QUEST FOR A BETTER BRAIN

Agnes Bediako Osafo-Gyimah (aka Afua Manu Oforiwah) RN, BSN.

ISBN 978-0-9976213-9-6 (paperback)

Dedication

To my granddaughters Megumi and Mari.
My daughters: Doris, Emi, Amma, Akosua Bediako and my niece
Mama Ofori-Kru.
My husband Professor Kwabena Osafo–Gyimah and my two sons,
Kwabena and Kwadwo Bediako.

ACKNOWLEDGEMENT

Evangelist Dr. E. A. Abboah-Offei: Grace Evangelistic
Center, Akuapem-Akropong
William Ameka: Manager *of Patmos Retreat Center*
Kwabena S. Owora
Rev. Doctor Daniel Nyanteh
My Pastor: Rev. Dr. Moses Biney
Neurologist: Dr. Carlisle St. Martin, MD.
Family Doctor: Dr. Albert M. Wright, MD.F.R.C.S. (C)
FACS. PC
General Surgery and Vascular Surgery.
My Nephew: Kwame Frempong, BSN, CRNA

My Niece: Akua Frempong

Contents

Foreword

Every effort in this book has been made to ensure that the information about the brain is complete and accurate. However, neither the publisher nor the author is capable of rendering professional advice or service to any reader. The ideas and suggestions contained in this book are not intended as a substitute for consultation with your physician. Individual readers must assume responsibility for their own safety, medical health and well-being. Neither the author nor publisher shall be liable or responsible for any alleged damage arising from any information or suggestion in this book.

Introduction

Rev. Nyanteh and I attend the same church, Bethel Presbyterian Reformed Church of Brooklyn. He talked to the whole church about the New York Theological Seminary (NYTS) one Sunday in 2008. I registered for admission the same year and it was at the school that one of my professors told me to consider writing. I shall forever be grateful to Rev. Dr. Nyanteh.

I retired in 2007 and therefore it was good for me to go back to school again. I suppose it was because I had reached a stage in my Christian life where I was still searching for knowledge about my calling and my Christian Faith. Although I had reached my retirement age, I still felt there was something I needed to accomplish even though I couldn't figure it out then.

In 2008, my husband and I watched one Dr. Daniel Amen on PBS (Public Broadcasting Station) Television. The topic was on his book, "*Change Your Brain, Change Your Life* ". This was the year after my retirement from working as a registered nurse in the Post-Anesthesia Care Unit (PACU) at New York Methodist Hospital in Brooklyn. After my husband and I listened to Dr. Daniel Amen on PBS in 2008, I decided to seek help. So **we** wrote to Dr. Amen via email, requesting for evaluation at his clinic. We were disappointed to find out that the clinic would not take our medical insurance (Medicare). We would have to pay cash and the cost being so much, we asked if there were any grants or senior citizen discounts. Unfortunately, we were told none was available. We gave up the idea but continued to subscribe to his newsletters via email.

I celebrated my seventieth birthday in 2011 and I started searching again, as that "*still, small voice*" in me kept telling me that something was not right. This same year I enrolled in a community school in Brooklyn trying to be computer savvy, however, I felt I was not retaining what was being taught. This was about the third or fourth time that I had tried to learn about computers.

The "*not remembering things*" had become worse, therefore my search began again. About the same time I watched Dr. Amen on PBS again and this time the topic was, "Use Your Brain to Change Your Life", another book he had written. After listening to him the second time I wanted to have a better brain to change my life, hence **my quest for a better brain,** which led me to being diagnosed with a large unruptured brain aneurysm. This book is about how it all unfolded.

What is the brain?

The human brain is involved in everything we do. It is that by which we move, live and have our being. Our decisions or reactions are all controlled by the brain. As a Christian, I love when the Bible said, "In God we live, move and have our being" (Acts 17:28a).

The brain is an organ of soft nervous tissue contained in the skull of vertebrates. The brain functions as the coordinating center for all sensations, intellectual and nervous activities of the body, according to Oxford dictionary (www.oxforddictionaries.com/us/definitions/AmericanEng lish/brain).

Today, many people, and especially many scientists, have different definitions about what the brain is and what it is not. We will talk more about the brain later.

CHAPTER 1

My Illness: How It All Began

I n 2011, my husband and I listened, for the second time, to a talk on PBS by a brain psychiatrist, Dr. Daniel Amen. The topic was "Use your brain to change your life". The talk was about the human brain and how the brain changes as one gets older. Dr. Amen talked about how one can slowly improve or even reverse the aging process. The first time we listened to him was in 2008 when he had talked about "Change Your Brain, Change Your Life". We bought at least six copies of his book and distributed some to friends and family. We also listened to the audio tapes included in the books.

One thing he said that resonated with my husband and I was, "psychiatry is the only medical field in which the doctors treat the patient without looking at the organ they are treating". We all know that in psychiatry one talks to the doctor and he or she prescribes medication. This, to me, was so very true. In Doctor Amen's recent YouTube video, he says "it's like throwing darts in the dark on a dart board."

Dr. Daniel Amen, M.D. and the Amen Clinic

Dr. Amen is a clinical neuroscientist, a child and adolescent psychiatrist. He is the medical director of the famous, internationally known, Amen Clinic for Behavioral Medicine in Fairfield, California. Dr. Amen is the recipient of awards from the American Psychiatric Association, the Baltimore-D.C. Institute for Psychoanalysis, and the U.S. Army. Dr. Amen is a nationally recognized expert on the relationship between the brain and behavior and on attention deficit disorder. He is an expert on brain image scan called SPECT *(Single, Photon, Emission and Computerized Tomography)*. SPECT is a nuclear medicine study that is used by psychiatrists to help diagnose their patients. It is also a study that is used to detect all kinds of brain tumors and cancer. SPECT tells the psychiatrists about activities in the brain - whether the activity is good or bad, too little or too much. SPECT shows the brain's blood flow, and most importantly, the shape of one's brain. Dr. Amen showed scans of some patients according to their chief complaints, habits, lifestyle, age etc. I thank God that with SPECT, psychiatrists get to look at the organ they are treating.

During the lecture Dr. Amen showed different kinds of brain scans and the effects of illness on them. He talked about and showed scans of healthy brains and diseased brains and how we can use brain health to improve our age. He recommended that one should have one's brain tested to get a baseline of one's brain.

My husband and I couldn't help it. We fell in love with his talk. We were so impressed that the very next day, in 2008, we called the Amen Clinic. We wanted to know if I could be examined at the clinic. I had this strong feeling after listening to him that his clinic could help me with my forgetfulness. When we called, we were surprised how much the secretary said it would cost to get a complete evaluation at the clinic. My husband and I are both retirees, so we wanted to know if the clinic accepts Medicare insurance or if there was any discount available for senior citizens, but the clinic had none.

We decided to forget the idea for the time being. However, in my quiet times, the "*still, small voice*" kept on telling me that something was not right. We both continued to subscribe to Dr. Amen's newsletters via email. We kept in touch and waited for God's time.

Dr. Amen used himself as an example by showing his brain scan when he was thirty and when he was fifty–it's unbelievable how remarkable the difference is. It was amazing what exercise, good diet and good habits did for his brain. His fiftieth year brain scan looked healthier than the thirtieth because he had been out of medical school, away from its stress of not sleeping and coffee drinking. Dr. Amen talked about how having poor memory alone can be a number one sign that one's brain is struggling. He said Alzheimer can start 30-50 years in the brain before it shows itself later.

So, I knew, at 67 plus years of age, that my brain was struggling. However, I gave up the idea of going to the clinic as result of how much it cost for an initial assessment. But l did not give up on being "*Brain Envy*" as Dr. Amen puts it; the hunger of wanting to know about my brain health continued. So, here I am in 2013, a couple of years later, a student in a community school; trying to learn more about the internet. I came home one day in February 2013 and told my husband that I was not going back to the school after the spring break. I told him I didn't think I was learning anything and added that maybe "I really need to see Dr. Amen after all". The next thing I knew, my husband went upstairs and came back down to tell me he had made an appointment for me to see Dr. Amen. That was a shocker! It was Wednesday afternoon and I was traveling to London the next Saturday. I asked him how much the fee was this time and he responded, "Listen, this is your health. I don't care if we have to get a bank loan." He was also told Dr. Amen does not see patients anymore; he only does research, therefore I would only get to see an associate in the New York office.

Dr. Albert Wright, M.D.

My doctor, friend and mentor is the one and only Honorable Dr. Albert Wright, M.D. A board certified, general surgeon specialized in vascular surgery, with an infinite patience for his patients. He is so caring that all his patients say, "He is a friend". I know this because I worked with him for about 23 years and had the opportunity to talk to and listen to his patients as their nurse. He is the one and only MD friend of my family. To talk about him and his kindness I need to write another book. He is an angel. There are not too many physicians like him left in today's world. Thursday, the next day, my husband and I decided to talk to our family doctor. The Amen Clinic had said we had till Friday evening to confirm the Monday appointment when my husband called.

Dr. Wright's office hours are Wednesdays and Fridays, from 5p.m. till the last patient leaves. His setting is "walk in, first come, first seen" basis. So we walked in at about 6 p.m. on Friday (three o'clock Pacific time). Dr. Amen's clinic appointments were made California time and the secretary had asked us to call to confirm before 5 p.m. We had told Dr. Wright about our intentions for me to see an award-winning psychiatrist and how we were going to spend money we did not have at the time. We told had him we must confirm a Monday appointment before eight o'clock Friday, New York time, which is five o'clock California time.

This evening he just listened as my husband and I went into his office and when I told him I thought something was wrong with my brain, he smiled. My doctor and friend has this healing, uplifting, comforting and charming smile that no matter how frightened or worried you are, when you step into his office, you start to heal. That is spiritual and angelic, isn't it? Yes! There is something angelic and spiritual about him. At least that is how I always feel and I know I am not alone in this respect. His patients are always saying complimentary things about him as they wait to see him. It is for this rare, tender and loving care that patients will wait hours to see him.

As usual he asked how long it's been going on. He said he had not noticed any unusual changes in me. However, he added that since I felt that way, we must do an MRI of the head since a thorough search revealed none on my file and if something was wrong then we would take it from there. He did not judge or belittle how I was feeling, neither did he brush my suspicions aside. He promised he would refer me to a neurologist that would take my medical insurance, therefore I should not worry. Immediately he picked up the phone and called the hospital for me to do an MRI of the head the next day. That is my doctor friend; he does not waste time. He listens to his patients and acts accordingly. I had my MRI done Saturday morning as scheduled at 10 a.m., had a normal weekend and went back into the office Wednesday evening. I could tell all was not well when I walked into his office and saw the expression on his face that Wednesday evening. I did not see that angelic smile. Maybe it was because it had been an unusually hectic day for him in the hospital. There were many patients waiting in the office to see him and he came in late, close to 7 p.m., instead of the usual 4 or 5 p.m.

He did not alarm me, but simply said "Well, Agnes, the report says there is atrophy and calcification somewhere in your brain, therefore I am going to refer you to my friend, the neurologist that I told you about". He put my radiology report in an envelope, sealed it and wrote the doctor's name and telephone number at the back of the envelope and gave it to me. He told me the doctor's office was in Queens and asked me to call the next morning to make an appointment. We were out of his office in a jiffy. On our way home, I was driving and was talking to my husband when I said, "Well, atrophy at age 71 years plus, not bad. Anyway, I'll schedule the appointment to go see the doctor for when I come back from London." I was not scared. I was my jolly old self, happy that nothing serious was found other than atrophy and calcification.

Chapter 2

Thursday Morning: The Wakeup Call

I was ready for school when I decided to call Dr. St. Martins' office and make an appointment with the secretary for one month's time when I would return from my trip to London for a vacation. A male voice answered the phone and asked who had referred me. When I told him that Dr. Albert Wright had referred me, he asked me to open the envelope and read to him the impressions on the report. I did so and his response was that he would like to see me now, today! He said he could see me in his office in Queens at 11 a.m. or in Manhattan at 3 p.m. First of all, I was expecting an answering machine or an answering service on the other end when I made the call. I did not know it was the doctor himself who was on the other end. He mentioned his name when he answered the phone, but I forgot by the time he finished telling me what to do.

Dr. Carlisle St. Martin

Dr. St. Martin was a one of a kind Queens, Forest Hills, New York, neurologist and family practitioner. He was so dedicated that I later learned that he was practically married to the office. I responded, "I am only calling to make an appointment for one month from now because I'm traveling out of the country next Saturday for a month." He replied. 'No! Mom! You are not going anywhere. I need to see you today!'

At this time I had begun to panic, so I said "doctor... (I tried to remember his name). Now you're going to make me cry". He responded jokingly, with a great sense of humor, "you better cry at home than in my office because I will not have tissue papers for you in the office. I would like you to go and get the CD of the MRI from where you had the test done and bring both the report and CD with you. I can see you in the Queens office or in the Manhattan office." My husband and I decided to see him in the Manhattan office. We drove to pick up the CD from the radiology center. Funny enough, though I was crying, it did not sink in how seriously ill I was. This was in February, now it is July and I have not driven my car since. Suddenly, unsteady gait, poor balancing and fear had taken control of me and for that the family would not allow me to drive. Maybe it's because of the way everyone in the family pampers me since the diagnosis. I am treated as if I am an egg that one has to be careful not to break. How can my life change so dramatically, so quickly, so suddenly, so drastically? I was not prepared for this at all. In fact, it happened just overnight! Last night I was happy driving from Dr. Wright's office with my husband by my side and today I cannot believe what has happened. A new dawn, with its mysteries! However, I knew even then that God was in charge. I was no longer crying when I got to the radiology place to pick up the CD, but I just couldn't believe the events of the morning. I picked up the CD from the radiology department, drove back home, prepared brunch for my husband and me, and after eating, we left for Manhattan by train.

Trip to Manhattan

Before my husband and I left the house we searched Google for information about Dr. Carlisle St. Martin and many positive things were said about the Forest Hills Queens doctor, a neurological brain scientist whose clientele was mostly Jewish. A dedicated, all trusting doctor whose friendship was cherished by his patients. Dr. Carl St. Martin is another angel, according to all the testimonies about him on the net. I just knew I was in good hands.

As mentioned before, everything seemed so unreal after I spoke to Dr. Carl St. Martin in the morning. We arrived at the Manhattan office at 2 o'clock for a 3 o'clock appointment. My doctor was on time. He came in at about 2:45p.m. with his assistant. In fact my husband and I asked each other "was that the doctor who just walked in?" They both said Hello!, but one of them, the one we saw on the Internet was on sneakers, with a dressed shirt and tie on; very neat but casual for Manhattan, I thought. That was the first time I had seen a doctor outside the operating room area with sneakers on, so I wondered and said to my husband "he truly must be a very down to earth person".

He came back outside with his assistant, introduced them both and gave us an iPod to complete all questions. He said it was a new way that he was admitting patients, without a secretary; and without doing face to face interview for that process. He said we could call his assistant if we had any difficulty. Of course my husband, being a computer expert, did all the work. The admission process was completed and the doctor called my husband and I into his office at exactly 3p.m. Dr. Carl St Martin welcomed us in such a friendly manner and acted most of the time like there was nothing serious to worry about. In fact he said I might be able to travel to London as planned. Dr. Carl St. Martin seated us comfortably in the office and took the CD of the MRI and the referral from Dr. Albert Wright from us. He commented on how well he knows Dr. Albert Wright. He said their relationship went far back as when he, Dr. Carlisle St. Martin, started his medical residency in Brooklyn at Downstate Hospital. He said he couldn't have gone through his residency without the kindness and the support of Dr. Albert Wright. He had so many good things to say about Dr. Albert Wright. Then he commented on Dr. Wright's gorgeous handwriting. All three of us agreed that Dr. Wright has the most authentic, charming and beautiful handwriting for a doctor; among nurses, doctors have the most illegible handwriting of the establishment. I thank God for the computers of today, as nurses can now read doctor's orders with ease. He added that Dr. Wright is one dedicated MD that he knows. His office hours are from 5 p.m. to whenever the last patient leaves, yet he had to make hospital rounds and sometimes had seven o'clock in the morning OR schedule in the hospitals. We agreed Dr. Wright is one of a kind. He said people say that he, Dr. St. Carl Martin, is very devoted to his practice, but there is none like my doctor friend, Dr. Albert Wright.

We knew everything Dr. Carl St Martin was saying about himself was the truth because that was written about him on the Internet. I told him my husband and I agreed to everything he was saying about my doctor and friend. In my mind I said here is a pot calling the kettle black. I added that my husband, Dr. Wright and I grew up together in the same town, Cape Coast, in Ghana. It was an instant bonding with Dr. Carl St. Martin.

Dr. Carl St. Martin put the CD in his computer and started to explain the different sections of the brain and how my abnormality was. He reassured me that everything was alright and that I might even be able to go on with my trip to London. Then he added that the CD was not too clear and therefore he would like a repeated MRI and an MRA at a radiology center in Manhattan. The MRA with contrast would give a clearer vision. My London trip will depend on the outcome of both he said. He gave me an eye and ear examination before sending us to the radiology place on 61st St., Park Ave in Manhattan. He asked us how and by what mode we came to his office and we told him we came by train. He took us to the reception area and faxed the referral to the radiology place on Park Avenue, followed by a phone call and told us to take a taxi cab there.

The time was about 4:30 p.m. when we got into a yellow cab on 42nd St. 10th Ave. to go to the 61st St. on Park Avenue Radiology, NYC. When we got there at about 5p.m. the receptionist called this lady who came and insisted to pay for the taxi fare because Dr. Carl St. Martin wanted her to do so. She wouldn't take no for an answer. My husband and I could not understand why. I have never heard of a doctor paying for a patient's transportation without the patient expressing that he or she could not afford to pay. I guess I would never know why such kindness, so I took the money and we were directed to the ground floor level where my test was to take place.

Chapter 3

The Experience at the Radiology Place

A technician introduced himself to us and properly identified me. He told me all was ready for me, took me inside and assisted me into the MRI machine, ear plugs and all. I was in the machine for about ten minutes when the machine stopped and I was assisted outside. I thought the first part was completed and that unlike the other radiology place, it took ten minutes instead of twenty. No one said anything to me and I did not ask any questions. One thing, I knew for sure that the MRI of the head takes about twenty minutes, just like the first one I did in Brooklyn. Next, they let me sit inside and a technician tried to start an IV on me in the arm. I was told it was for the MRA.

The IV was a difficult prick; the technician could not find a vein on either hand. I thought it was because he was not experienced enough, but he called for a second and a third person who equally tried, but it was in vain. Finally, after I suggested should put the small butterfly needle at the back of my left hand, a vein was located and the IV was started. Then I was asked to wait, followed by a couple of phone calls to and fro by the technicians. Some time passed and a technician who came to put the contrast checked my order again and spoke to someone upstairs.

Then the technician put me back in the machine with my IV in place, but clipped off. I was in the machine for about twenty minutes this time. I was taken out of the machine and eventually the technician took out the IV and said I was done for the day. The time was about 7 p.m. when I left the basement to go upstairs. The secretary at the desk told me she had been waiting for me to reschedule me for another test in the morning.

I became confused and told her I had two tests done downstairs. She explained to me that they stopped the first time because my insurance company will not pay if they do two tests the same day. I was shocked to hear that, I was not aware that such a thing exists in America today with insurance companies. Then again, the technician downstairs did not bother to explain anything to me. I called Dr. Carl St. Martin who had earlier told me to give him a call anytime the tests were finished. He was very understanding and told me to make an early morning appointment for the next day, Friday, February 8. As such, I made the appointment for 9a.m. and took a taxi home alone because my husband had left earlier for his evening computer class at the same adult community center that I had been going to. He had a final exam so he left the radiology center a few minutes before seven to make it to his class by eight o'clock.

Friday, February 8th, 2013. The weather forecast for Friday, February 8th, 2013, was a prediction of this big snowstorm for the New York/New Jersey area and the whole east coast. The poor weather forecast was to start anytime in the afternoon. My husband and I left the house Friday morning at 7a.m. to Manhattan via taxi for my 9a.m. radiology appointment; this time my daughter took the day off to go with us. We arrived early for my nine o'clock appointment and were taken in right away. My test was completed by 10 o'clock in the morning. My doctor had instructed them to give me the CD of both tests, the one from the previous day and that of today. He also told us to call his office for further instructions when everything was completed.

Weill Cornell Presbyterian Hospital

Dr. Carl St. Martin told us when we called that he had seen the report from the Park Avenue radiology place and that the result was as he suspected. He instructed us to take a taxi to go to Weill Cornell Presbyterian Hospital on York Avenue, between 1st Ave. and 68th Street. He gave us a doctor's name to ask for when we get there. We were directed to the doctor's suite and were told he was in surgery and therefore we should wait because he had been expecting us. He came shortly after and saw the film and told us that he had referred us to another doctor because his specialty was on the human spine. This, by the way, is the brain and spine unit. Weill Cornell has a huge building for brain and spine surgery. I saw it for the first time that day.

Dr. Philip Stieg, the chief of surgery for the brain unit was also in the operating room and he too was going to see us shortly. Dr. Stieg's assistant interviewed and prepared me to complete the consultation form. Dr. Stieg made us feel at home and he explained everything on the CD to us in a layman's terms. He made a sketch of the aneurysm, how large it was and where it was in my brain. He ordered further tests;

a blood test for cholesterol and a CAT scan of the head, contrasts too needed to be done immediately and then we should come back to his office. The whole process took about one hour to be completed. Unfortunately for us, when we got back, we were told the doctor had a family emergency and had left the hospital for the weekend or until further notice. We were told that his nurse practitioner would call or get back to us. Who says the devil is not alive? Well, God is more alive and powerful; He began it and he will accomplish it! Halleluiah!

We called Dr. Carlisle St. Martin from Dr. Stieg's office at Weill Cornell and he told us not to worry. He said he had been faxed the report of the CAT scan and that he would have a conference call with us at the comfort of our house at 8p.m. He told my daughter how to set up her computer for the conference call. So we left the hospital and came home without further ado because of the predicted poor weather. Modern technology was or is fantastic. They had predicted heavy rain and storm after the rush hour, so Dr. St. Martin warned us to get home on time to get ready for our conference, which we did over Skype with Dr. Carl St. Martin. Dr. Carl St. Martin patiently explained to all three of us what needed to be done; he also advised me to cancel my scheduled trip to London the next day, the day of the predicted heavy snow and rain, February 8, 2013. Cancellation was easy because all international and domestic flights were suspended because of the snowstorm. I was given a whole year to rebook my flight.

Chapter 4

The Diagnosing of an Unruptured Brain Aneurysm

My family and I visited Dr. Carl St. Martin's office in Queens on Sunday. He examined me physically and went over all my medical reports. He said "Yes, all the findings were in and I have a large unruptured brain aneurysm with calcification." The calcification meant that the aneurysm has been there a long time and no one can say how long. Given the size of it, I have been lucky that it never ruptured.

The brain

The brain is an organ that controls all the various organs and systems in the body. The brain is an organ of soft nervous tissues contained in the skull of vertebrates as I said in the introduction.

The scientific study of the brain and nervous system is called neuroscience or neurobiology. But what is the human brain? To me the brain is the mover, the maker and the shaker of the body; the engine of the body and soul.

The brain is the coordinating center of all sensation, intellect and of nervous activity, according to National Institute of Health (NIH, April 28, 2014). It is the 3.3lb organ which is the center of intelligence. The brain is the interpreter of the senses, initiator of body movement and the controller of behavior. The brain is the source of all the qualities that define our humanity. It is the crown jewel of the human body. In nursing schools, in-service trainings and modern neuroscience seminars, one is taught about the brain, but nothing compares to the free information on the internet.

The brain lies in its bony shell and it is washed by its protective fluid- the blood-brain barrier flow. The human brain is the largest among all vertebrates. It is about 2% of our body weight. It contains billions of nerve cells called neurons connected by billions of connections or synapses. The cerebrum, which makes most of the brain's weight, is the gray matter and it contains billions of nerve fibers (axons and dendrites), forming the gray matter.

Until recently, scientists knew very little about the functions of the human brain, just about 10% of what the brain does. However, there has been so much advancement in brain research and development in the last five years. Today I joined a poll on the internet about sending campaign message reminders to my congress to make September a brain awareness month.

In April 2013, one month after my surgery, President Obama and his cabinet voted $100 million dollars towards brain research. A lot is happening about the brain today. My mission is to make awareness of brain aneurysm and its devastating effect on the family, and already we have won an effort for the nation to dedicate a whole month to brain awareness. Wow! God is really in control, working behind the scenes and looking out for us. Some intellectuals say the brain is like the universe, the galaxies; while others even say the brain is the God in us. In Genesis 2:7, during creation God put his breath in man and man became a living being-the only creature in God's creation that received God's breath.

Shakespeare says the brain is the sacred dwelling place of the soul and as a Christian, my Bible, throughout history, talks about the *soul* as God's sacred dwelling place. Personally, I believe the soul is the breath we take. Therefore, my brain is my essence, my whole being, who and what I am and ever will be. If my brain is not functioning well, it means I am truly not well. My brain is the engine of my body, my being, my breath, my soul and my spirit.

So, this is the moment I started questioning and talking to my God. What now, my Lord? Why now? You have brought me this far, now what? Ok, Father, I know you are in control. Thine will be done, oh God my savior. The saying that man proposes, but God disposes came to mind. Here am I today with so much on my mind and yesterday I had very little to worry about. But one consolation was that I knew God was in charge and that all would be well. So at that moment I surrendered it all to God and started singing the third verse from my Reform Church hymnal #302, "Have Thine Own Way, Lord", asking God to take control and to heal me.

Brain Aneurysm

A brain aneurysm, also referred to as cerebral aneurysm (CA) or intracranial aneurysm (IA), is a bulging weak area in the wall of any of the arteries or blood vessels that supply blood to the brain. This weakened, widened or abnormal ballooning spot on an artery or vein is a risk for rupture or bursting. It often looks like a berry hanging on a stem. Some describe it as a balloon-like blister that forms on an artery. Others say it is a weak or thin spot on a vein or artery in the brain that balloons out under high pressure and fills with blood. Whatever they call it, it is a very serious and life-threatening illness when it ruptures. Blood to the brain is food to the brain. Food to the brain means life. Without good nourishment to the brain, life is short of proper existence. The bulging or ballooning in the blood vessel exerts pressure on the walls of the artery and if one is not lucky the wall breaks and blood leaks into the brain. In the lucky ones, meaning the patients who are lucky, the berries stay small, asymptomatic, with or without calcification, and no breaking or leaking manifest itself. According to Dr. J. J. Jaffa (the doctor I saw for consultation at NYU), many people go to their graves with aneurysms. The estimate is that some six million Americans live with unruptured brain aneurysm. Sometimes the pressure causes slow leakage onto the brain, which too can cause stroke or mini stroke. The brain matter is gray and blood leaking onto it is like a dark cloud over the skies, causing obscurity, which is unacceptable. This dark cloud over the brain makes everything black instead of gray or white, thus making everything redundant. One cannot think straight or function properly. Where there is light would be darkness and where one could see before, one could be blind. Not a pretty sight, I must say!

There are two types of aneurysm: saccular and fusiform.

Saccular

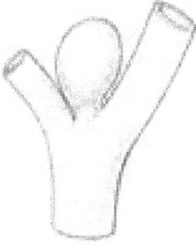

A saccular aneurysm is the most common type of aneurysm and accounts for 80% to 90% of all intracranial aneurysms, according to National Brain Aneurysm Foundation/glossary. They are the most common cause of non-traumatic subarachnoid hemorrhage (SAH). It is also known as the "berry" aneurysm because of its shape. It looks like a sac or berry forming at the bifurcation or the "Y" segment of arteries. It has a neck and stem. These small, berry-like projections occur at arterial bifurcations and branches of the large arteries at the base of the brain, known as the Circle of Willis.

Fusiform

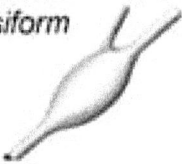

The fusiform aneurysm is a less common type of aneurysm. It looks like an out pouching of an arterial wall on both sides of the artery or like a blood vessel that is expanded in all directions. The fusiform aneurysm does not have a stem and it seldom ruptures.

What is a Brain Aneurysm?

A brain aneurysm is a weak bulging spot on the wall of a brain artery, very much like a thin balloon or weak spot on an inner tube as described earlier.

According to the Brain Aneurysm Foundation, 1 in 50 people have a brain aneurysm and about 40% of people who have will die - very, very serious! Therefore one has to take the warning signs/symptoms serious.

Warning Signs/Symptoms

Unruptured Brain Aneurysm

Some warning signs and symptoms are: localized headache, dilated pupils, blurred or double vision, pain above or behind eye, weakness and numbness and difficulty speaking. Most of the above, I have been experiencing for years and I had no clue what they were.

Seek medical attention immediately if you are experiencing some or all of these symptoms!

Some risk factors that doctor and researchers believe contribute to the formation of brain aneurysms are: smoking, high blood pressure or hypertension, congenital - resulting from inborn abnormality in artery wall, age over 40, gender - women have an increased incidence ratio of 3:2 relative to men, and finally family history of brain aneurysms - which is my portion among others. Most questionnaires given at the neurologists' offices are geared to reveal above signs/symptoms and risk factors, yet there is not much education after one completes these questionnaires.

Bleeding within the brain tissue itself is called intracerebral hemorrhage and it is usually caused by complications of hypertension with an aneurysm rupture. We have already established that the brain controls the body, therefore all systems could go wrong or down with the rupture of an aneurysm. Depending on what area of the brain was affected and how much of the brain was affected, a whole part of the body it controls could be affected. The usual outcome is that 30-40% of victims of ruptured brain aneurysm die. And the other 60% suffer malfunctioning. Some cannot talk, see, walk, and perform activities of daily living. They have to be assisted in eating, putting on their clothes, ambulating etcetera; majority become tremendous burden on their families. It is very devastating to both the patient and their family when this happens. As a nurse, I took care of patients who had suffered strokes and just the simple act of saying something can be so frustrating when words cannot come out right. Watching and seeing the effort they have to put into every step they take, whether it is in eating, walking, clothing themselves, or talking was very difficult for me. So one can imagine how their loved ones feel.

In some cases an aneurysm may leak a slight amount of blood. This leaking (sentinel bleeding) may cause extreme and sudden extremely severe headache. A more severe rupture almost always follows this leaking. First we will talk about unruptured brain aneurysm, which is what I had.

Unruptured Brain Aneurysm

An unruptured brain aneurysm is an aneurysm that has not yet ruptured. Its presence may not be known most of the time until it ruptures or is accidentally discovered through a routine checkup for another illness. My case was discovered, as I explained earlier, not through a routine checkup, but through my personal intuition that something was not right and I therefore went to my doctor for help. How many of us get that chance? How often do we listen to our intuition, the still, small voice in us telling us good things to do?

How is Brain Aneurysm Diagnosed?

Based on my experience or the process I went through, the following tests are usually performed by the doctor if they believe or suspect you have a brain aneurysm:

A computed tomography (CT) scan can help identify bleeding in the brain if one has ruptured brain aneurysm with subarachnoid hemorrhage.

Computed Tomography Angiogram (CTA) scan uses a combination of CT scanning material (dye) injected into the blood to produce enhanced images of blood vessels– remember my radiology experience. Magnetic Resonance Angiogram (MRA) is similar to CTA. MRA uses magnetic field and pulses of radio wave energy to provide angiography; a dye is often used during MRA to make the blood vessels show up more clearly. For Cerebral Angiogram (CA), during this x-ray test a catheter is inserted through blood vessels in the groin or arm and moved high up to the blood vessel in the brain. A dye is injected into the cerebral or brain arteries. As with the above test, the dye allows any problem in the brain to be clearly seen on the x-ray.

Although CA is more invasive and carries more risk than the two above, it is the best way to detect small (less than 5 mm) aneurysms.

How it is treated

Your doctor will think of several things before deciding on what course of action for treatment is best for you. Treatment determinants would include already discoursed parameters such as age, overall health, size of aneurysm and any additional risk factors. Your doctor may want to continue to observe your condition rather than recommend a surgery because the risk of small aneurysms (less than 10 mm) rupturing is low and surgery is often risky. Some of the following surgeries are used to treat both ruptured and unruptured brain aneurysm.

Embolization

A small tube is inserted into the affected artery and positioned near the aneurysm. For **coil embolization**, soft metal coils are then moved through the tube into the aneurysm, filling it and making it less likely to rupture.

In **mesh embolization,** a mesh is placed in the aneurysm, reducing further blood flow to the aneurysm, making it less likely to rupture. These two are less invasive and are believed to be safer than surgical clipping.

Surgical clipping

This surgery involves placing a small metal clip around the base of the aneurysm to isolate it from normal blood circulation. This decreases the pressure on the aneurysm, thus preventing it from rupturing. Some aneurysms bulge out in such a way that it has to be cut off and the end of the blood vessels stitched together, but they say this is very rare. Sometimes the artery is not long enough to stitch together and a piece of another artery has to be used. Aneurysms that have bled are very serious. In many cases they lead to death or disability as I have said before. Management includes hospitalization, intensive care to relieve pressure in the brain, maintenance of breathing and vital functions (such as blood pressure) and treatment to prevent re-bleeding (WebMD Medical Reference from health wise. January 03, 2013). Not all brain aneurysms rupture and doctors are now able to detect unruptured brain aneurysms with an increased frequency because of the growing availability of non-invasive imaging methods such as an MRI/MRA that patients are more comfortable with. An unruptured brain aneurysm may or may not give symptoms. As opposed to ruptured aneurysms which require urgent treatment in almost all cases, unruptured aneurysms may require treatment or may be followed with serial imaging studies in some cases.

Things doctors consider in deciding whether or not to treat an unruptured aneurysm

Like ruptured aneurysms, unruptured aneurysms may be treated with either endovascular coiling or open surgical clipping. However, if the unruptured aneurysm is treated successfully, the recovery period is generally shorter than that of a successfully treated ruptured aneurysm. Although survivors of unruptured brain aneurysm treatment may suffer many of the same physical and emotional symptoms as a survivor of a rupture, they will have a shorter hospital stay, require less rehabilitative therapy, and return to work more quickly.

Symptoms of an unruptured brain aneurysm

Symptoms include but are not limited to the following: headaches*, dizziness, blurred vision or vision difficulty (problems seeing), eye pain: drooping heaviness of eyes or tired eyes. Also, forgetfulness, neck pain or neck tension and fatigue. I have lived with the above symptoms for most of my adult life. I had no idea. My purpose for this book is to make my readers aware about these signs/symptoms. Talk to your doctors if you feel or have felt any of these symptoms. Other symptoms include numbness, weakness or paralysis of (often) one side of the face, and seizures. If an aneurysm is small, it may produce no symptoms. Most documentations say so, but as I said earlier, I have felt the above symptoms most of my adult life and I cannot prove at what size or age the symptoms appeared, and neither can the doctors, so for now my advice is that if there is a family history of strokes, get tested once you hit age 40.

A large unruptured aneurysm may press on brain tissues and nerves, possibly causing pain, especially above and behind an eye. It may also cause dilated pupil, change in vision or blurred vision, sensitivity to light, and drooping eyelids.

*Seek immediate action if you experience or develop extremely severe headache.
Call 911 or your local emergency number.

Risk factors that doctors and researchers believe can cause or contribute to the formation of brain aneurysm: Smoking, high blood pressure or hypertension, family history of brain aneurysm, congenital i.e. resulting from inborn abnormality in the arterial wall. Ages over 40, gender— women have an increased incidence of aneurysm at a ratio of 3:2 compared with men; drug use, particularly cocaine, infection, and tumors and traumatic head injuries.

Risk factors that doctors and researchers believe contribute to the rupture of brain aneurysms: Smoking, high blood pressure or hypertension as result of thinning and degenerating arterial walls, often at the point where the arteries fork, bifurcates or branches off - these points are the natural pressure points of a vein or an artery, and are easily the weakest link in any blood vessel. Although aneurysm can appear anywhere in the brain, they are most commonly found in the arteries at the base of the brain. Risk factors that develop over time are numerous, some are more common in women than men and attack more blacks than white; it also attacks more adults than children, older people age being the most at risk. Other risk factors that could lead to the development of aneurysms over time are smoking, high blood pressure (hypertension), hardening of the arteries (arteriosclerosis), drug abuse, heavy alcohol consumption, head injury, and certain blood infections, as well as lower estrogen levels – as is the case postmenopausal and in diabetic patients. Family history of brain aneurysm is also a factor, particularly if a first degree relative such as a parent, a brother or sister suffers from one as I already stated.

Polycystic kidney disease, an inherited disorder that results in fluid-filled sacs in the kidney and usually causes increased blood pressure is also a risk factor.

What causes an unruptured brain aneurysm to bleed or leak?

High blood pressure: This is the number one silent killer and we must do all we can to prevent or control its onset. Diet, exercise, lifestyle and good habits can play a part in the prevention of this terrible illness.

Strong emotions: Such as being upset, angry or overexcitement are not good. It is good to be calm always. Smiling is healthy and is a good therapy for the brain.

Blood thinners: Such as warfarin, as well as some medications or drugs e.g. cocaine.

Cost

The financial cost of aneurysms is huge, especially when the cost to insurance company and the family are considered. Medication and equipment cost is skyrocketing. However, the cost is nothing compared to if it is not detected on time, that is why creating the awareness is very important. A cane I needed after my surgery for steady gait cost me twenty eight dollars and that was not the most expensive one on the shelf. The cost for rehabilitation can be prohibitive; who can put a price on patient and family suffering?

Signs and symptoms of bleeding (hemorrhagic stroke): Sudden severe headache, nausea and vomiting, seizure, drowsiness, and/or coma. The following may also be present:
A) Weakness or paralysis of arm or leg.
B) Difficulty speaking or understanding language, and
C) Vision problems.
(American Heart Association Inc. Feb. 2013)

Ruptured Brain Aneurysm

Ruptured brain aneurysms usually result in a subarachnoid hemorrhage (SAH), which is defined as bleeding into the subarachnoid space. When blood escapes into the space around the brain, it can cause sudden symptoms such as: severe headache, loss of consciousness, changes in mental awareness or orientation, seizure, nausea/vomiting, stiff neck, sudden eye pain or difficulty seeing.

If brain aneurysm ruptures, it releases blood into the skull and causes stroke. Ruptured brain aneurysm is called subarachnoid hemorrhage. Depending on severity of hemorrhage, brain damage or death may occur. The most common location for brain aneurysm is in the network of blood vessels located at the base of the brain called the circle of Willis (WebMD. 2005-2014).

Signs and symptoms of rupture

Common signs and symptoms include sudden and extremely severe headache, nausea and vomiting, stiff neck, blurred or double vision, sensitivity to light, seizure, a drooping eyelid, and Confusion (May 23, 2014. Mayoclinic.com).

"Many people live with brain aneurysm and take it to their graves" says Dr. Jaffa, the neurologist I consulted for a second opinion. Dr. Stieg already explained to me before I went for the MRA that there seems to be calcium formation with the weak arterial bulging in my brain. This would be an indication that it had been there for a long time. Normally he would say that I should not worry, but the size of what was there, 14mm, indicated that action needed to be taken. He said that it could be left alone, but the size of the aneurysm would be the indicator whether I needed surgery or not, and the CT scan ordered would help to determine or confirm the size.

Dr. Carl St. Martin also said when we visited him in his office on the Sunday, that with my young age and given the size of the aneurysm, he too recommends that I do something about it, to prevent future rupture and possible stroke. Dr. Carl St. Martin assured us that Dr. Stein's nurse will call us and make the necessary appointment soon. He confirmed that the doctor had a family emergency and will not be in the office the whole of the following week. Dr. Carl St. Martin reassured us I will be in safe hands and that I had nothing to fear or worry about. I was more relaxed when we left his office. I had no fear at that moment.

Chapter 5

The Wait

Waiting for a brain surgeon to call was a week of torture for me. The weather was so bad, the snowstorm came and international flights to and fro JFK were cancelled. It was very easy for me to tell my ailing sister in London that my flight had been cancelled because of the weather, and that I will reschedule as soon as possible. But what do I tell my second family, the Church members who keep calling the house to find out if I was able to make my trip or not because of the weather? My husband was assigned to answer the phone calls and tell everybody that called that my flight wasn't able to take off as planned. My sister in London was getting better so I told her I will have to reschedule my flight and that will take time. Lying to my church sisters and brothers over here was the hardest part.

One week went by and I did not hear from Dr. Stieg's nurse. Finally I called the office during the second week and the nurse told me they were trying to arrange with the interventional radiologist who will perform the procedure to come from his two weeks' vacation. Dr. Stieg wanted to wait for an appropriate time that the radiologist, himself and my family could meet to schedule the appointment. They called back to assure me that they were planning for my family to meet the two doctors at the same time and that the second doctor would also be available in two weeks' time. This was a very trying moment for me. Waiting was hard but I had no choice. God's word says we should watch and pray plus give thanks, and that is what I did. For the next two weeks I stayed at home with my husband and daughter catering for all my physical needs to reduce my stress. This is the time that my daughter arranged for me to have a second opinion consultation at NYU with a top-notch brain neurologist, Dr. Jaffa who confirmed the findings from Weill Cornell and said that he would follow the same course of treatment. In fact Dr. Jaffa said he knows the interventional radiologist at Cornell that we have been waiting to see. He said the route Dr. Stieg has taken was the best; he would have taken the same route.

I did a lot of research on the Internet myself. We all did, especially my daughter who is also an RN. There is so much information on the Internet about brain aneurysm which I did not know existed. I learnt one is not born with brain aneurysm, yet one can inherit it from a first degree family member. If a mother or father dies of a stroke or suffers from a stroke, chances are a brother or sister will have a stroke, according to AHA. This, I cannot stress or emphasize enough.

My mission to bring the awareness: Why?

My mother died of stroke in 1983 in Ghana. She walked into the hospital complaining of diarrhea, nausea and vomiting. The only treatment she received was IV fluids for hydration. She was in the hospital for twenty four hours. Back then I am sure the doctor did not have the equipment and tests to help them diagnose aneurysms. My sister who was with her was told she could take our mother home the next day. When she came for discharge the next day my sister was told our mother passed away during the night. Just like that! She did not become sick for even one week for us to pamper and nurture her a bit. Her death took all six of us by surprise, but then that is what a brain attack does.

Tia or Stroke

The cause of death as noted on my mother's death certificate was stroke, or a TIA (transient ischemic attack), a condition that occurs when blood flow through an artery that supplies blood to a portion of the brain or the heart is blocked and therefore there is restricted blood flow to that area of the organ. So I thought my mother died of heart attack all these years. Blood supplies oxygen-rich food to the brain. Without that there is no good health of the brain. The brain controls everything the body does, therefore lack of proper nourishment to any area of the brain is a distaste to the body. My first MRI report said there was some atrophy of some blood vessels and calcification. Later, after surgery, my doctor confirms that I have had several mini strokes. If only I had the information that I could inherit brain aneurysm from a parent, I would have had an MRI much earlier. Maybe the several mini strokes could have been prevented. This is why I must proclaim the awareness of the disease and its hereditary component. Everyone should be aware and do an early screening and testing plus follow up. Maybe soon all the insurance companies will pay for MRI of the head and it will become a routine test, just like screening of the breast - mammogram. I would not have lost so much of my memory as a result of having several mini strokes. I would have had an MRI of the head done as far back as in the eighties when my mother died. Two of my biological sisters have had mini strokes. I also have a brother who I suspect have suffered several mini strokes. My brother and his wife are both scheduled for MRI of the head. This is too close for comfort for my family, four out of six is huge; where is the awareness? My brother and sisters who have already been diagnosed with strokes all live in different countries or states. So, environment has nothing to do with this illness. Nevertheless, I have made it my mission post-procedure to make people aware about this devastating illness, brain aneurysm; the genetic component factor is my biggest emphasis. It also attacks more female than men-in my family, the ratio is 3:1.

Race: More blacks than white.
Previous aneurysm: People who have had a brain aneurysm are more likely to have another attack.
High blood pressure: The risk is higher in people with a history of high blood pressure. I fall into the above categories don't I? So my body has been talking to me all this time. How I walked into my doctor's office and told him I think there is something wrong with my mind, is amazing, mind bothering and by God's intervention only. I know it was all God's Grace. Also, Dr. Wright did not doubt me nor brushed me off. He took me serious and took action right away. God was at work behind the scenes on my behalf and I thank Him for that. The speed with which Dr. Wright acted was amazing. He normally would write a referral to be taken to the lab, but

this time he picked up the phone, made the appointment himself and then wrote the referral. I know God is alive. How else was that possible? This also means we should pay attention to what the small, little voice in us whispers to us always.

Chapter 6

The Genetic Component

The genetic component of brain aneurysm needs to be understood. Somehow, until now, I thought my mother had a heart attack because of the 'TIA' on the death certificate. I didn't know and I never connected her death to me until now. I did not know my mother died of brain attack, despite having worked in the medical field all my life. My hospital where I worked and retired from and where I worked for more than twenty three years was not specialized in brain surgery. I am yet to learn that even in America today, one could die if one is taken to the wrong hospital during an attack; and there are so few hospitals specialized in brain surgery. They have specialties for hospitals and for every part of the body. This is true of all the organs in the body. So how come there is only few hospitals in the city specialized for the controller of the body? Nevertheless, many of the best brain hospitals are in NYC, Manhattan. Three of the best are right here in Manhattan. There is Weill Cornell, NYU and Columbia Presbyterian Hospital (CPH). Such information is easy to find on the Internet and is very essential. I learnt in 2015 that NYMH and CPH have joined together and now NYMH conducts the same procedure I had done in Manhattan in 2013. NYMH in Brooklyn is saving lives daily with this procedure.

This waiting period is when I learnt so much about the brain on the Internet and on the television. Drs. Rudy Tanzi & Deepak Chopra gave a talk again on PBS about "The Super Brain: How to Turn Your Mind into A Super Brain." The talk discussed how we are not our brains, but the user of our brains. Dr. Tanzi talked about the different parts of the brain and their functions in the body. What effect or part food and good diet plays; and what part poor dietary habits and illness plays. He explained the reptilian brain, the instinctive (the body) brain, the limbic (the spirit) brain, the emotional brain and the neocortex (the mind) i.e. the reasoning brain with such fun. He is a great actor just like Dr. Daniel Amen.

Dr. Deepak Chopra was a bonus in this talk with his enchanting meditative voice about exercises, diet and good living advice. Thanks to Oprah/Deepak, this was also the first time I joined the twenty one day meditation on OWN. I thank God for all the blessings thrown or showered on me at this trying period. The most devastating news at this time was when I had all my three biological children tested with an MRI of the brain since it is noninvasive. Fortunately for me, none of my children smoke. None had drug abuse problems or history of alcohol abuse. All three were above thirty five years of age, with no history of hypertension or high cholesterol.

Yet, one tested positive for a brain aneurysm, a size of which two opinions recommended surgery. One can only imagine my guilt and devastation with this report. The fact that I could have passed this history on to my child. However, God is good! At least now the family is aware. The first two doctors recommended surgery, whilst the third doctor recommended observation. And so we continue to pray for the power, the anointing power of God, to do God's Healing. I have faith and hope in God's power. God is our "Jehovah Rapha," our healer God. Amen!

What Is Stroke?

According to the National Institute of Heart, Lung and Blood Associations:

> A stroke occurs if the flow of oxygen-rich blood to a portion of the brain is blocked. Without oxygen, brain cells start to die after few minutes. Sudden bleeding in the brain can cause a stroke if it damages brain cells. If brain cells die or are damaged because of a stroke, symptoms occur in the parts of the body that these brain cells control. Examples of stroke symptoms include sudden weakness; paralysis or numbness of the face, arms, or legs (paralysis is an inability to move); trouble speaking or understanding speech; and trouble seeing. A stroke is a serious medical condition that requires immediate emergency care. A stroke can cause lasting brain damage, long-term disability, or even death. If you think you or someone else is having a stroke, call 9–1–1 right away. Do not drive to the hospital or let someone else drive you. Call an ambulance so that medical personnel can begin life-saving treatment on the way to the emergency room. During a stroke, every minute counts.

Ischemic Stroke

An ischemic stroke occurs if an artery that supplies

oxygen-rich blood to the brain becomes blocked. Blood clots often cause the blockages that lead to ischemic strokes.

Hemorrhagic Stroke

A hemorrhagic stroke occurs if an artery in the brain leaks blood or ruptures (breaks open). The pressure from the leaked blood damages brain cells. High blood pressure and aneurysms are examples of conditions that can cause hemorrhagic strokes. (Aneurysms are balloon-like bulges in an artery that can stretch and burst.) Aneurysms exert pressure on the part of the brain where they are.

TIA or Mini Stroke

Another condition that's similar to a stroke is a transient ischemic attack, also called a TIA or "mini stroke." A TIA occurs if blood flow to a portion of the brain is blocked only for a short time. Thus, damage to the brain cells isn't permanent (lasting). (This I am not so sure of. I was told the first time I saw Dr. Athos Patsalides that with brain aneurysm whatever I have lost in memory before the procedure may not come back. This he said was due to "mini strokes". Dr. Patsalides found out during my procedure that I have suffered several mini strokes. I asked how many and he said he did not count them. Like ischemic strokes, TIAs often are caused by blood clots. Although TIAs are not full-blown strokes, they greatly increase the risk of having a major stroke. If you have a TIA, it's important for your doctor to find the cause so you can take steps to prevent a major stroke.

Both strokes and TIAs require emergency care.

Researchers continue to study the causes and risk factors for stroke. They're also finding new and better treatments and new ways to help the brain repair itself after a stroke

Stroke is the #1 leading cause of death in the United States according to the National Stroke Association. It is also the number 1 cause of long term disability. Many factors can raise your risk of having a stroke as I have talked about. Talk with your doctor about how you can control these risk factors and help prevent a stroke. If you have a stroke, prompt treatment can reduce damage to your brain and help you avoid lasting disabilities. Prompt treatment may also help prevent another stroke (www.webmd.co/brain aneurysm).

Chapter 7

Diet

P oor eating habits, such as consuming foods high in white sugars, white flour, high carbohydrate, low protein and high wrong fat diets is generally not healthy. Also, eating too much at a time or having unbalanced diet is not healthy either. Instead, we need to eat the right foods, small portions at a time.

My Background

I worked as a dietitian in two New York City Hospitals for fifteen years.

Training and Work Experience

Food Service: Firstly, I went to school at Hadassah University, Israel in 1965. I had an FAO scholarship to train as a Nutrition Extension officer. I worked as such at Korle Bu Teaching Hospital, Accra, Ghana, 1966-1968 before coming to the United States of America. In the USA, I was hired and worked as a dietitian in the Jewish Memorial Hospital, Manhattan from 1968-1979. During this time I took causes in diet and nutrition at Hunter College Manhattan and I also worked at Logan Memorial Hospital from 1979-1981. These years, 1979-1981, were some of the years of former Mayor Koch of New York City, during which time he and his administration decided to close certain hospitals in Manhattan. Jewish Memorial hospital, which had declared chapter eleven and was near bankruptcy in 1978 was one of them. Again that was my cue, a turning point for me to move on and perhaps find a profession in which there would be more job security, flexibility and satisfaction; a profession in which I would continue to have daily contact with patients.

As a dietitian I had daily contact with the hospital staff, with patients through checking of the daily menus, supervision of kitchen employees, distribution and serving of meals, ordering of food for the hospital etc. My hospitals had a system of putting menus on the patient's breakfast tray and the dietitian making rounds before lunch to collect and check them; making sure their requests have been properly circled and that each patient was following their diet as prescribed by the doctor plus having a balanced diet. The dietitian was seen by each patient Monday through Friday to answer their questions; discuss menus and educate patient and family plus give them a chance to ask questions. This part of the daily activities of the dietitian was what I loved and enjoyed most. I had the same feeling as a nutrition extension officer at the outpatient clinic at the Korle Bu Children's Center, Ghana, where I used to talk to pregnant and lactating mothers about food and nutrition. The teacher in me manifested and this was gratifying.

Logan Hospital was marked as one of the hospitals to be closed in Manhattan by Mayor Koch and his governor. Among their arguments was the proximity of Logan and St. Luke hospitals. They said the two hospitals were too close to one another and Logan hospital, being a community hospital, was not large enough and was not bringing in enough money. I started looking for the same job in other hospitals when my hospital declared chapter eleven. To my surprise they wanted a degree or master's degree for the position I held for more than eleven years with a diploma. So I decided to either change my major or to go into nursing, for flexibility of schedule for my family and personal satisfaction. The money and benefits were almost the same because most hospitals were unionized those days. Unfortunately, both the two hospitals I worked in closed in the 1980s. As such I am tempted to say a little bit about nutrition and brain healthy foods.

Brain healthy diet or foods come from:
Leafy greens: for example kale, spinach, dandelion (these three plus walnuts and half of an apple is my favorite morning slush or smoothies), collard green, broccoli, Brussels sprout, parsley, chard and all other greens and colorful leafy vegetables, as well as every herb. (Color is important: chlorophyll is good for the intestinal lining, among other things).

Cauliflower, beets, red or green cabbage, and red or white onions are very good; the darker the color, the better the nutritional value. Then there are the squash group, which includes acorn, bell and zucchini being my favorite.

Nuts and pulses: walnuts, almonds, peanuts; and pulses - beans, peas and legumes.

High protein foods: These include lean protein foods such as skinless chicken and turkey with extra fat off, fresh and dry fish, shellfish and lean beef and pork. This brings us to foods high in fats such as animal skin.

We will discuss parent essential oils (PEO) later.

Fruits: The saying that "an apple a day makes a man healthy and wise is not for nothing." However, berries, especially blueberries are my favorite, yummy! According to recent nutritional values, blueberries are among the number one super brain fruits. Fruits are better when eaten first thing in the morning, instead of when eaten as dessert or as snacks between meals. A fruit cup as the first meal in the morning, followed by water works like magic for bowel movement.

Condiments: Mushrooms, avocado, ginger, garlic, and all other condiments both fresh and dry. These are classical nutritionally; ginger and garlic are my main spices. Sage, basil, oregano, dill, mint, and all peppers are also my favorite. Hot peppers; Wow! Ghanaians love hot peppers, but we shall talk about this another time when we deal with recipes.

Whole grains, corn, brown rice, tubers, especially sweet potatoes, plantains (especially ripe plantains), but only in moderation. Ripe plantains, cocoyams, Malaga coco (brobe) and sweet potatoes have low glycemic indexes and are good for the diabetics. I tried it on my diabetic husband, friends and all diabetic family members and it has been proven they can eat a little bit more than the regular; but as said before, everything in moderation. Fantastic flavored chocolates or cocoa. Of course Ghana's history as an international producer of cocoa has a lot to do with my passion for chocolate. Ghanaians love chocolate and dark chocolate is one of the brain boosting foods; the best dessert ever. I wish Ghana will one day become a leading chocolate dessert country.

Milk: A necessary nutritional component, especially for growth, but a luxury food item in a country like Ghana where I was born and grew up. Only the rich can afford to drink milk or use milk products.

Tiger nuts: The good news is that the chief crop of my hometown for export or marketing is tiger nuts. The only cash crop in my hometown is still the growing of tiger nuts. Growing up, we ate a lot of tiger nuts. It was our main dessert and was either eaten raw (fresh) or cooked. We grew up on it and we did not know its nutritional value. Today, one can hardly afford it because they still use the old primitive method of farming to grow tiger nuts in Ghana; therefore the market is still tight. I hope "Graceland farms," with its modern machines will change this soon. My daughter sent me an article this year whereby Whole Foods in New York have tiger nuts on the shelves as an exotic nutritional organic dessert. I hope my hometown will wake up and make tiger nuts again its number one leading crop for export. The soil there is different and perfect for tiger nuts' growth. This is one of the areas where investors are needed for farming.

Tiger nuts have several essential nutritional food components that would be beneficial for infants, children and the general population of Ghana.

Thenationonlineng.net featured on all the social networks "Health benefits of tiger nuts". Another food for thought!

Oils: All the years I did nutrition education (1963-1968) in Ghana, the imported nutritional textbooks we used stated palm oils were the worst oils to use for cooking. That was and is still the most common oil to be found in Ghana. Peanut oil and coconut oil are Ghana's olive oil. Kernel oils are abundant in Ghana because palm nuts and coconuts were marked as not good for consumption because of their high saturated components. But now, in 2015, the PEO solution by Brian Scott Peskin (BSEE-MIT), says, they are the best oils for human consumption. According to him and his partner, so are animal fatty foods like the skins of chicken and other animals. They say these oils are conquering cancer, diabetes and heart diseases.

Check it out!
Drs. Stanley Jacobs, Ronald M. Lawrence and Martin Zucker talked in their joint book "The Miracle of MSM" about the natural solution for pain. Their book has been around since 1999, claiming relief of pain from headaches, muscle pain, arthritis, athletic injuries, allergies and more. MSN is a natural mineral solution. It stands for methylsulfonylmethane, a natural substance present in food and in the human body. An essential mineral oil, an amino acid, that practicing doctors

need to look into just as they need to check into PEO (Parent Essential Oils) solutions as mentioned earlier. Again, going back to basics via modern intervention can sometimes get frightening. I wonder if FAO has a special committee set up to go through all the different claims around today claiming that certain solutions and herbals are good for us; claiming that they can cure all kinds of diseases. Ghana today is saturated with herbal drinks and remedies. Everything and everyone has gone herbal, even beer, water and wine. This is where we need to operate with caution. Example is the use of noni fruits and leaves and also moringa. Ghanaians have been using these two plants lately with disregard to side effects. My fear is that too little knowledge can cause more harm than good, therefore we should use these herbals with caution.

Water - the best drink ever. A class of its own.
The human brain is made up of about 75% - 80% of
water.
- Dr. Joseph Mercola 1997-2016.

Herbs and some beverages: All herbs and spices, teas and other beverages (half a glass of red wine a day for dining if preferred) are healthy. Most of these are medicinal, but we don't know them. Our ancestors used them to treat all sorts of illness and most of them lived to be over one hundred years and more. Today, medicine has gone back to the basics. Dr. Oz has a concoction for gas using anise seeds, caraway, dill and fennel. It works and I use it as my anti-gas cocktail instead of the medication Nexium and Mylanta. The above foods are also heart healthy. All of the above foods, except leafy greens, can be used in moderation. One can go overboard with leafy greens for fullness, fiber and for important vitamins and mineral essential to the body.

Chapter 8

My Signs and Symptoms

Before my MRI of the brain, whenever I visited a radiology place, I had to complete a family history sheet. Similarly, each doctor I visited asked about family history. Stroke as cause of death for my mother was always documented on these sheets, but it never rang a bell until now! I had no clue why they asked us those questions and I don't know why no one ever explained the connection with a parent having a stroke and its relevance to their children and siblings. I mean the genetic component to stroke. The doctors and nurses gave no explanation as to why they wanted that information. I am a retired RN and I have worked in hospitals in NYC since 1968 yet I did not know this. An x-ray of the head somewhere on my medical chart for reference would have prevented a lot of irreversible damage to my brain that the doctors are claiming now. But God is good. I did not know and I thank God for the discovery now. It is all by His grace; God protected me all these years of mini strokes. Here is where I sang "My redeemer/To God be the glory" by Nicole C. Mullen. Amen!

Again an aneurysm is a balloon-like bulge of an artery that supplies oxygen and rich blood with nourishment to the brain. An aneurysm is abnormal. It can stretch and burst with devastating result. A brain aneurysm is caused by weakening of this balloon-like bulge of an artery that supplies oxygen-rich blood to the brain. The weakening causes a deviation of blood flow to the area, making a balloon-like bulge which, if it ruptures, can be fatal. Thus, strokes are caused by ruptured brain aneurysms. We all know the color of the brain is gray; some say white, and blood is red, therefore the two does not mix. Blood onto the gray matter is like a dark cloud over the sky. One's world is shut down. No more light where there was once light. There is no more sunshine, joy and harmony. Darkness takes over the whole body. Depending on what part of the brain is colored by the leak or rupture, a part of the body can become redundant, not belonging any more. Not part of the whole. Stroke is a terrible illness that we should do everything in our power to prevent. I think there had not been enough advocacies for its prevention. So I continue to hammer it in. Don't be overwhelmed by my repetition.

Gradual Memory Loss

Well, my symptoms so far had been a history of gradual memory loss, which I kept to myself, hypertension and borderline high cholesterol, neck tension and vision problems.

Vision: Reading

The problem with vision is recent. I never needed reading glasses until in my 40s. Before then, I had no problems with my vision. From September 2012 until the week of January 2013, I visited my eye doctor several times because I had blurred vision after reading for about 45 minutes. I had my glasses changed three times. I could tell my eye doctor, whom I have known for years, did not know what to do with me. Every time he turns around I was in the office complaining about my reading glasses. He actually sent me or referred me to another doctor; a contemporary, just for a second opinion to check my eyes and also to check my reading glasses. The second doctor said she was not going to refit me with any further reading glasses because what I have is the same as what she would have recommended. So this was the state I was in when I decided to get my head checked; a student who cannot read for about an hour before all becomes blurry and who cannot retain what she reads or learn. Go figure! Not a pretty sight! Not a good thing. However, having a blurry vision and neck pain or tension was two of the major signs of brain aneurysm, but these were never picked up by any of my doctors; because there has not been enough awareness in the past about brain aneurysm. Thanks be to God for the Internet! During the weeks that I was waiting for the doctors to get together and call me, I did a lot of research on the Internet about ruptured and unruptured brain aneurysm. I was amazed at all the information available out there. I had no idea. I read and listened to videos and audios by doctors till I knew what exactly they would be doing to me when the time comes. I learnt which hospitals are the best nationwide and how I was lucky to be living in NYC with several of the best right where I was. By the time I was called for my appointment with doctors Stieg and Athos Patsalides, I was an educated consumer with a second opinion under my belt.

I learnt a lot about brain aneurysm by googling the subject on the Internet. There were doctors from various hospitals and clinics readily explaining each procedure to give the patient confidence. Via the Internet, one is able to learn which hospitals are the leading ones. This gave me so much confidence that by the time I met with my doctors I knew what questions to ask and what answers to expect. Thank you WebMD/Mayo clinic/AHA and all the brain doctors on the Internet from the various hospitals. I searched and read most of what you had out there.

Sickle Cell Carrier

I have always suffered from mild headaches. The headaches have been with me all my life. I learnt when I was a teenager, that mild headaches are some of the signs and symptoms of having sickle cell traits; a circulation problem that gives chronic mild headache. Thus, I have learnt to deal with this by elevating both feet whenever my legs are tired or by lying down and taking short naps, even if it's five minutes, to improve circulation back to the heart. As a carrier of sickle cell, I always have bilateral feet and ankle pain and swelling while standing. I have learnt too that sitting and elevating my legs eliminate both the pain and the swelling, so that has been my only medication or remedy over the years.

Chapter 9

My Medical History

The MRA and the CAT scan I had done at Weill Cornell Presbyterian Hospital confirmed the aneurysm was large and therefore needed to be removed. It also had calcification all over it and I was told it meant that it had been there a long time. There had been no previous tests to compare so no one could say how long it had been that size or how long I have had the aneurysm.

Gastric Ulcers: I had my gastric ulcer under control by using Dr. Oz's anti-gas cocktail or papaya enzymes when needed.

Hypertension: I have had a history of high blood pressure for more than thirty years. Therefore, there is no telling how long I have had the aneurysm, but I suppose the hypertension was one of the causes. Maybe that was why I was able to stay calm and cool during the time I waited for the doctors to connect.

Thyroid problems: I have had thyroidectomy and have been on synthroid daily since 2009.

High cholesterol: I have had high cholesterol for about six years now. My doctors say I do not need any medication for control my cholesterol is controlled by diet only and my good cholesterol has been within normal limits since the past six months as confirmed by my lab work. Once my endocrinologist thought I needed to go on Statin drug for the cholesterol. She prescribed and I took it for about two months. I stopped it because I did not like the way it made me feel. Then my husband went on the Internet and Wow! There were so many negative things about Statin drugs. We think no one should take it. Again, this year the PEO solution book is saying cholesterol is one of the essential oils our bodies need. Our body will produce it if it needs it; so why mess it up with medication? There are other exacerbating causes of aneurysm such as diabetes, obesity, alcohol abuse and drug abuse and I thank God I have none of the above history.

Family History: My mother had a history of high blood pressure, thyroid problem (goiter) and sickle cell Anemia. I inherited sickle cell trait, hypertension and goiter from my mother. My endocrinologist requests blood works twice yearly to make sure my blood values are normal. I believe that how well one fares with surgery and recovery depends on one's state of health before the whole thing. In fact I had just done my semi-annual blood work for February and my values were all within normal limits therefore I did not have any repeated blood work for my surgery though the tests were done at different hospitals. I believe this is all the result of modern interventions and the computer. My lab report was faxed from the original hospital to the hospital where my procedure was to take place - from Brooklyn to Manhattan. Medical clearance report was faxed from the various doctors via phone calls without any reexamination by these doctors. This system eliminates unnecessary costs to both patients and the insurance companies.

Chapter 10

Consult At Weill Cornell
February 25, 2013.

Finally, the time came for me and my family to meet the two doctors at Weill Cornell Presbyterian Hospital. The date was February 25th, 2013. We met the interventional radiologist who was to perform my procedure. Dr. Athos Patsalides, who went over my history and my lab works, examined me and explained what was needed for the procedure. He asked if we had any questions; requests for medical clearance was sent to my family doctor. Cardiac clearance plus gastric clearance was also needed. The latter was because I have had a history of gastric ulcers and aspirin and Plavix would irritate the stomach. I needed to take both medications for ten days before the procedure. The medical clearance was easy. I have had all my doctor's checkup, including eye checkup just a month earlier, therefore all I had to do was to contact my various doctors and ask them to fax the reports to doctor Patsalides' office.

Tuesday March 12, 2013.
Blood Thinning Test

I was given my blood thinning medication prescription, so as soon as all my reports were in, I had a call from the nurse practitioner at Weill Cornell to start the meds and to report to the hospital lab on the seventh day for a special platelet blood count test. Tuesday March 12, 2013 was the seventh day of taking aspirin and Plavix as ordered. Thus, the day for my test was a lousy day. It was a rainy day and it was very windy at times during the day. I was asked to report to the lab at Weill Cornell at 11 a.m. They would have lab requisition ready at the desk for me. This was the day that so many incidents, including a miracle, happened. We arrived at the hospital on time for my appointment via taxi in the rain and reported to the lab. My papers were ready at the desk and they asked me to have a seat.

The Devil at Play

The technician called me shortly and said the hospital had a problem. The machine they use for the test, the only one in the hospital, was out of service that morning. She kept on apologizing, yet no one made an effort to call me about the problem before I left the house. I asked her what we were to do next and she replied that she didn't know. I asked her to call upstairs so that I could speak to the nurse. She did that and my nurse was just as surprised. She said she will talk to my doctor and get back to us. During my waiting period at the desk, another technician who overheard us and thought she knew the area well came to our aid. She told the clerk I could have the test done at the Quest Lab on 68th Street and York Avenue. I asked the clerk to call my nurse; she was glad for the information, and ask her to release my lab request form to me so I could go to the Quest Lab. Before she gave me the papers, I asked her to call the place first so that they would be expecting me. She appeared reluctant but she called and the phone rang for a long time with no one answering.

So she hung up and wrote the phone number at the back of the lab sheet before sending us on our way. Outside was rainy, windy, very gloomy and almost dark even though it was about 12:39 p.m. My husband and I had umbrellas so we started walking. One thing, the clerk did not give us the cross streets, just the avenues, and she added that the place was a walking distance. So we walked, York Avenue, First Avenue, Second Avenue and then Third Avenue before we reached the building. Our pants were soaked wet because of the wind factor. When we got there the technician took my requisition form, looked at it and told me they do not perform that test at the lab. In fact she called the office that would perform the actual test and was told that the special test needed to be performed as soon as the blood specimen is drawn. That is why the machine has to be at the premises.

This was a big disappointment. I was so upset I just had to sit down for a while. I called my nurse practitioner to tell her what was going on. She too was upset. She asked to call me back after she speaks to my doctor. She called back after a while and said my doctor says he can perform the procedure without the test and therefore I should go home. She said the test was only to confirm my blood bleeding levels and that his experience tells him that I shall be alright. I became more upset; I did not want to have a procedure done under such conditions. To me, not doing the test means selling myself short for such an important medical procedure in my life. Of course that did not resonate well with me and my family. But we had no choice but to come home. When God is within, all ends well (Se Nyame wo mu a biribiara bêye yiye).

Nyame wo mu o, wo muo,biribiara bêye yie.
Nyame wo muo bibiara bêye yie.dc
{Nyame wo muo, Nyame wo muo. }
{Biribiara bêye yie.}
Agya nyame wo mua biribiara bêye yie.
When God is in control, all will be well.

I sang this Ghanaian Gospel song the rest of the day.

Chapter 11

Intuition or Miracle?

Tuesday March 12, 2013, continued.

We got home about 3 o'clock in the afternoon. This is what I call the miracle of the day. I had an intuition to call New York Methodist Hospital and ask for the lab department to find out if they do that special test. Methodist is the hospital that I used to work at and I knew the number for the lab offhand. And what do you know; the lab receiving clerk that answered the phone on the other end was someone I knew! I asked if they do the test and whether their machine works and she answered yes! I also wanted to know if the test should be done at any specific time and she said I had until 7 p.m. that day. To me that was an intuition becoming a miracle, God was on my side. Thank you God!

We had a light lunch and my husband drove us to the New York Methodist Hospital. However, when we got there and after I registered, the technician told me that for almost a month they had not had the special butterfly needles that they use to do the test. A supervisor was called who made several phone calls to check other areas and units and truly there was none. My procedure at New York Cornell Hospital was scheduled for Friday, so the supervisor asked me to come back the next day, Wednesday because she knew the test does not take long to perform and she hoped that in the morning they would find the needles for the test.

The next day was Wednesday, February 13. My husband and I left the house early to be at the Methodist Hospital by 7 a.m. As usual, we were there before the technicians came in. I was number one to register. The technician told me she did not have the needle to draw the blood. I told her I was in the other lab last evening and that the supervisor told me to come to her this morning. I wanted to know if any note was left on my behalf because the supervisor promised she was going to look for the needles. The technician answered that nothing was left for me. I became so noticeably disappointed.

The Power of Prayer

Disappointed? Yes! But not hopelessly broken. I started praying. As a Christian, prayer should be the breath and the step I take, but it had never done that. However, today I prayed and my Lord heard me. The above intuition became a miracle and I knew God was on my side. I knew I was going to have the test done at the hospital that morning! Somehow I knew God had already answered my prayer. Amen! The technician made a couple of phone calls and the next thing I knew she came to me and asked me to register and wait. She continued making more phone calls. I was number one of only four patients and the others waited patiently while she stayed on the phone. Eventually, she told me she was going to get the needles from upstairs. In just a few minutes she came back with a full box of these precious needles that the hospital has been waiting for months to get. Now, that was the power of prayer! My test was completed by 8 a.m. so my husband and I had breakfast at New York

Methodist Hospital that morning. I became relaxed. It reminded me of the times I used to work there and would go downstairs for breakfast when times permit. Having breakfast with my husband after twenty four hours of stress was a treat and very relaxing. Somehow the whole atmosphere was peaceful and even romantic. I have never had breakfast with my husband at the workplace. This eventually became one of the happiest mornings since I was diagnosed with brain aneurysm. I thank God for that moment. It was good! Somehow I was ready for surgery.

Oprah/Deepak 21-day Meditation

The week of March 10, 2013 was a very special week. It was the National Nutrition Week and New York Methodist Hospital was celebrating it at the atrium of the hospital on the first floor. My husband and I joined the class after breakfast at the hospital cafeteria. This was also the week that Ms. Oprah Winfrey and Dr. Deepak Chopra started their 21-day free meditation on OWN. It was the third day and I was so excited about the meditation because it was my first time joining. That too was the first time I learnt to meditate. A very big step I took with my daughter Amma as my encourager. At least 10 of my former coworkers that I met at the atrium knew nothing about the OWN meditation program and they were so happy when I gave them the contact to register. That made my day because Oprah/Deepak Chopra had already covered intuition and this is how far intuition had gotten me that day. I couldn't contain my happiness. I was elated and ecstatic! My husband kept on telling people we met that I had become an advocate for Oprah Winfrey/Deepak Chopra. I felt great because my test was completed and that meant in the afternoon I could call Weill Cornell Hospital for the exact time I would be reporting to the hospital for my surgery Friday morning. That also meant that I would go in for surgery with everything I needed to have a perfect surgery and recovery. I thanked God that I listened to that 'still, small voice' in me, my "intuition." I knew too that I was that calm because of the meditation. I completed the whole 21-day meditation with Oprah and Dr. Deepak, which was fantastic! You should see me pre- and post-procedure in the hospital. I had my iPod by my pillow. I kept the daily meditation playing on and on and on. Everyone that came into contact with me was told about the 21-day meditation. This was March 15th and 16th 2013, my hospital stay period.

Bethel Church and their First
40 days Easter Fasting

My church goes online every morning at 5 a.m. for Bible study and prayers. We use a free conference line for this. As many as one hundred people can dial in at any given morning to talk, pray and listen plus study the Bible. My church had started a 40-day fasting for Easter in January 2013. We usually do one week, two weeks or one month Easter fasting, but this time we did a whole 40 days fasting. My alarm comes on each day at 4 a.m. to prepare for my morning devotion with my church. I did not vigorously participate in the fasting part this year because of my history of gastric ulcers and the fact that I was on several medications. However, this year I decided to give up tea, juices, sodas and all beverages for the forty days. The only drink for me was water, warm or cold. I also cut down on my food intake and its portions. Therefore, the 21-day meditation starting March 11 was a bonus. I thank God for modern technology such as free conference calls and those who make it available for us. I lost at least five pounds and felt much better at the end of the forty days, which was a bonus in itself. Thank you Lord!

Boost of Energy

After the blood work in the hospital my husband and I went food shopping. I had so much energy. After all, my test had been completed, which meant I would be going in for surgery fully prepared with everything I needed. My daughter called while we were in the grocery store and told me that the doctor's office had not received the lab report yet. She could not understand why I was doing grocery shopping when I should be home resting in preparation for my surgery. I told her to relax and that I will call the hospital when I get back to the house. I told her that God was in control and that she should stop worrying. I have noticed for some time now that she hovers over me like a mother over her defenseless child. We were home by 2 p.m. and I called the lab, gave my date of birth and the technician said that in five minutes my doctor in Manhattan will have that report in his office. The office called me at 4 p.m. and the nurse practitioner told me everything was set for Friday morning. That I should report to the hospital at 6:30 a.m. with my family. She gave me my pre-operation instructions on the phone. She told me that I would be a DOSA (day of surgery

admission). She also called my daughter and gave her the
same information plus the directions and the area to report
to at the hospital. Thursday was uneventful. I stayed at home
all day just taking it easy. Morning Bible study/prayer by my
church plus the daily 21-day meditation with Oprah/Deepak
which comes on my email every morning at 3.15 a.m. were
all I could do. I had my last meal between 6 and 7 p.m. We
also made taxi arrangement for 5.15 a.m. pickup. My bag and
clothing was packed and ready for the morning.

Chapter 12

The Day of the Surgery: March 15, 2013

The Taxi Ride

Friday March 15, was the D-day. I woke up at 3 a.m., took my shower, dressed up and did my 21-day meditation with Oprah and Deepak Chopra. The car service was downstairs exactly at 5:20 a.m. and we were on our way. Little did we know that Brooklyn Bridge was closed at that time every night until 6 a.m., but God was on our side. The cab driver we had that morning knew how to maneuver his way around. I had confidence that all will be well so I was in a relaxed mood the whole trip. We arrived at Weill Cornell Presbyterian Hospital surgery unit at exactly 6:15 a.m. The unit was very nice, quiet and neat. It was difficult to get to, but my daughter had the instructions packed. We were the only people there at the waiting area the time we reported. My chart was there and the receptionist asked us to have a seat. We were there for about thirty minutes before we were called inside to the recovery room area. I liked the set up. I was given a bed in the recovery room, curtains were pulled for privacy and I was instructed to change my clothes in preparation for surgery. My husband and daughter were with me in the recovery room all along. After I changed, my family was given chairs at the bedside and was told they could stay. I couldn't have asked for anything better or more. Shortly after we settled my nurse came, introduced herself and started the pre-op admissions.

She did my vitals, connected me to the EKG monitor and drew some blood as well. After the nurse completed her checklist, the anesthesia resident came with his consent forms for me to sign and explained that I would be given general anesthesia. I was also seen by the anesthesiologist who would put me to sleep. My doctor, Dr. Patsalides, also came and talked to me and the family. Everyone was very professional and assuring. I was very grateful. I was very calm because I knew my God was going to see me safely through this one too. There were other surgical team members who came to see me. I was scheduled for nine o'clock but my doctor came to inform me there would be a thirty minutes delay as result of an earlier emergency case going.

The Surgery

I was wheeled to the OR (operation room) via the recovery room bed. There were at least eight staff members that I counted in the OR who came to my bedside. My doctor and the anesthesiologist were there. Their assistants, nurses and some operating room technicians all came to introduce themselves. The bed was aligned to the operating table and I was asked if I could move over to the operation table, which I did. A nurse introduced herself and said she was going to insert a Foley catheter to my bladder and at the same time, the anesthesiologist applied facial mask with oxygen and asked me to start counting down from one hundred.

Extubation in PACU

I don't know how far I got counting, but I woke up with my bed now in the recovery room, with the endotracheal tube still in my throat killing me. A ventilator was in place.

The clock in my room read 2:30 p.m. Both my arms were restrained to the bed and the mouthpiece (the endotracheal tube stabilizer) was pressing against my pallet and that was what was killing me. In fact that was my only painful experience throughout the whole ordeal. I think it was wrongly positioned. It was pressing on my palate instead of my tongue. It hurt so bad I just knew it was wrongly placed. I started fighting and struggling right away and that made it difficult for me to breathe. I felt I was choking and the ventilator started backing off. My daughter was there and witnessed me struggling to talk, requesting to be extubated. She called the doctor who came right away. I was instantly extubated and placed on nasal cannula 3 liters/milliliters of oxygen. My attendant came to see me and congratulated me, saying that everything went as explained pre-op. He said the base of the aneurysm was too wide so they did not use a coil. Instead they did embolization by clipping. He also told me he found out that I have had several mini strokes. When I asked him how many he said he did not count them. The mini strokes were a surprise to me. When! How! No wonder sometimes my words don't come out as I want them to be. Apart from the forgetfulness and mild headaches, I have noticed for some years that my words sometimes do not come out right, but I never associated that with strokes. I loved my God more than I have ever done that instant, that moment when the doctor told me about the mini strokes. My God had protected me so much so that I didn't feel any of these strokes come on. What an awesome God. I started singing a song of thanks and praises to God and I did not stop singing all evening. I was so appreciative of my family

71

and of the hospital staff. I was happy to be alive.

My song was a Gospel one:
'What shall I say unto the Lord?
All that I have to say is thank you Lord'.

I loved the world more; I mean God's creation. I loved my family more. My heart was so full of joy, love, grace and gratitude. I thanked everyone that came near my bed. I was so happy to be alive and well. I cannot begin to tell how elated and happy I was whenever the doctors and nurses came to my bedside and assessed me for bleeding and also to do my neurological checks. God is good! Amen! I also sang the song:

God, you are so good, so kind, my lord, you are excellent.

My throat was hurting and very dry after the extubation, so the nurse supplied cotton swabs with mouth wash that my daughter applied periodically to my lips. It tasted so good. Again the throat pain was the only pain that I experienced post-op. I had my iPod and earphone with me so I listened to Oprah/Deepak 21-day meditation from day one. This was Day Five and I cannot tell you how helpful, comforting and consoling a role that had already played in my recovery. I felt like the whole program was made just for me. The first day talked about wellness, the brain and how proper diet and good habit is essential. I cannot thank you enough, Oprah and Dr. Deepak Chopra. My family stayed until about 9 p.m. I was able to tolerate water and jello for dinner. I had to be fed in bed because I had to lie flat on my back. The jello tasted like file meg yon! I had more than one jello. It soothed my throat pain. That, the water and the mouth swabs did the trick. I received one visitor. A very, unexpected, special visitor since my immediate family were the only ones I thought was aware of me being in the hospital. My pastor's wife, Mrs. Paulina Atiemo came to visit. I had called her on Thursday morning at 6 a.m. after our morning devotion and told her I never travelled to London because of my situation and that I was scheduled for surgery the next morning. She told me her husband was out of town and prayed for my successful surgery and speedy recovery. I was very appreciative for her visit. I was not expecting her to come all the way from Queens to Manhattan to visit me. I did not think anyone had the address of where my surgery was taking place except the two family members at my bedside. Mama Atiemo's visit was a big surprise. Moreover, she came by train and at the rush hour, between 4-5 p.m. She prayed for me and I, in turn introduced her to the 21-day meditation. None of the nurses at the unit knew about the free 21-day meditation so I continued my advocacy. I was more excited than ever! Here am I, alive and well plus I had no pain and was joyful.

I wanted the world to have and feel joy. Mama Atiemo left after 7 p.m. She wanted to leave after the rush hour. My daughter and my husband left my bedside after 9 p.m. and ordered me to try and go to sleep. My daughter commanded, "Mom, you have not slept since you woke up at 2 p.m. We are leaving. Just close your eyes even if you are not sleepy and

The Day of the Surgery: March 15, 2013.

you will fall asleep". I listened to my daughter, closed my eyes and told myself I am going to have a conversation with my maker, my God.

Chapter 13

Conversations with God

March 16, 2013: The adventure post-op.

I started praying, just thanking God for everything. I was so happy and just full of thanks, praise and adorations. All I could say at the beginning was, "Thank you Lord!" repeatedly. Then I started counting my blessings. My family, the nuclear family, and the extended family. My achievements. I was just so, so much full of gratitude. I thought about my friends and then my church family. I realized that I have been so blessed. 11:00 p.m. came and I was still awake and still praying or meditating, just talking to my maker, God. That was very unusual for me; I usually fall asleep within thirty minutes when I close my eyes to pray when I am lying down.

This night was different and the fact that I have had general anesthesia earlier even surprised me more because I have had several surgeries with general anesthesia and I usually fall in and out of sleep the first twenty four hours. Normally after general anesthesia I would spend the rest of the day dozing in and out of sleep. I turned my head to the left side with my eyes closed. Still talking to God, I felt a black hole or rather saw a big black hole inside of which was a white light which eventually takes over the black hole. This continued over and over and over like the Milky Way or moving clouds. I became concerned and even thought maybe I should not position my head on the left side since my surgery was on the left side of the head. I turned my head to the right side, with the rest of my body still dorsal (on my back) on the bed. That was not so comfortable. I repositioned the head of my bed up a little and soon the nurse came and put the head of my bed down as before, explaining that putting my head up that way will exert pressure on the groin and that is not good for me now. The Milky Wave continued even with my head on the right side so I positioned my head flat on my back and it stopped.

Encounter with the Spirit

Flat on my back with my eyes closed and still praying or having a conversation with my maker, I felt the presence of a Spirit descend on the left side of my bed towards the head. I became frightened at first. However, I had the courage and the presence of mind to say to the spirit, "You may stay if you are a good spirit from God, else I command you to go back where you came from if you are not the Holy Spirit of God!" This spirit was in the form of a person. I couldn't turn further enough to look at the face because I was flat on my back. Actually, the more I turned my head to the left side, the further away the Spirit moved. Therefore, I cannot truthfully give the accurate description of His face or the crown on His head. All that I can say is that the person had on a triangular shaped greenish tunic print. The tunic was aqua green. The spirit was also holding a triangular iron bar with metal chains around it in His right hand. I didn't know the significance of the triangle with the chains at the time, but weeks later some Catholic friends paid me a home visit and after I talked to them about the visions and added that I do not understand the significance of the iron tripod with the chains, they told me it signifies God the Father, God the Son and God the Holy Spirit.

The three in one – the Trinity, how awesome! What my friends, one from Jamaica and two from Nigeria, said made a lot of sense. By the way these are my friends that I co-starred with in the Nigerian film "Ma George" in 2012. Just one year before this illness, I was a movie Star. My Hollywood friends' visit was a big surprise and very spiritual. One of them, Ebo Ngwenya, called and said, "We are coming to visit if you would be up to it," and they were in my house in an hour. They brought their hymnals, sang gospel songs and prayed for me. The tripod as the three in one truly made sense. I never doubted the spirit in my visions, however my friends' explanation of the tripod greatly confirmed, strengthened and reassured me that God was with me all those hours.

After I told the spirit that He may stay if He was from God, I stopped being afraid. And the spirit stayed with me talking to me all night. I continued with my prayers and talked to the Spirit the rest of the night. My nurse kept on checking on me and repositioning me in hope that that would make me fall asleep, but all to no avail. I had no pain and somehow I enjoyed the company of the Spirit. The Spirit worked by drawing and even though the beginning of almost all the drawings did not make sense, the final products were familiar and beautiful.

Chapter 14

The Designer

I named the Spirit, "The designer". My husband and I own this plot in Ghana. We started building on it about two years ago. The main house is not yet completed and we still have a lot to go before its completion, then the extension or guest house is to follow. The Spirit brought me to the plot in Ghana and I recalled a day two years earlier when I invited my friend in the Lord, the powerful evangelist and prophet, Dr. Abboah Offei. That day he and his wife came to pray over the land before we started building (this is something Christians do in Ghana sometimes).

This incident was more than two years ago at the time of the vision. I recalled that my evangelist friend prayed, "Lord we thank you for Auntie Aggie's life; this woman who has decided to do things for your Glory, and to help others." I don't know if everybody that had gathered there that day heard him say that, but I did and in my mind, at that time, I said, but this is for my private abode only. At that time, I wondered why my evangelist friend said that I was building for others to enjoy. However, and interestingly enough, six month prior to that date, my husband and I were discussing the extension to the main house and I suggested that we make it into a bed and breakfast unit. Wow! Where did that come from? My husband strongly opposed the idea and said emphatically that the place will be for our private use only and that was the end of the discussion. So tonight the Spirit revisiting the scene with me made me wonder why. But then, who am I to question God's plan. I already said God is in control.

What is a vision?

Edith Wharton says "a vision is a manifestation to the senses of something immaterial. She says look not at visions, but at realities."

A vision is an experience of seeing someone or something in a dream or a supernatural manifestation or apparition. Webster dictionary defines a vision as a supernatural appearance that conveys a revelation, unusual discernment or foresight, a direct mystical awareness of the supernatural, usually in visible form.

I like Webster's definition. It portrays vision as the act or power of seeing. "With vision, nothing shall be impossible." (Tam Seth Eyedoude JP, May, 25, 2014).

The definitions go on and on and on. There are all types of visions, business, religious, inspirational etc. I think for now and since I will give you, my reader, how it all started, we will rely on our faith to guide us as to what a vision and mission is.

What is a mission?

In my case, the definition of a mission is to carry out humanitarian work; to sacrifice or give up something for the benefit of mankind. Per the Webster dictionary, a mission is a specific task with which a person or a group is charged, a calling - the work that a person does or should be doing. "Vision is where you are going, mission is the means you will use to go - how you will reach the destination where your vision awaits." (Apostle Daniel Kwakye, August 8, 2014).

According to www.derby.anglican.org/attachments, a mission is a word that is often used, but it is not easy to a find definition or meaning everyone agrees with. The above site has five definitions of mission and the fifth one is my favorite because that was my commission. A mission is to strive to safeguard the integrity of creation and sustain and renew the life of the earth. This is deep, for many have died trying. However, God always sees His visions to fruitful accomplishment. With all of the above said, we will venture into my spiritual adventure post-procedure.

Spiritual Adventure Post-procedure
The visions of the designer

I was in my hospital bed with my eyes closed, awake, alert, oriented and responsive, when the Spirit, the designer, takes me to a site, my new home at Peduase, Accra, Ghana. The designer started drawing. I could not or did not understand the pictures. He just continued to draw. The images were not clear at the beginning, but the drawings went on and on and on and 'voila!' there was a tall building in black and white, the white being the light's reflection inside the building. This building was huge! There was a beautiful flowery garden surrounding it at the base and it looked like a big hotel. I talked to the designer throughout the drawing. At this time I said, "But how? There is not enough space for a hotel where we are building at Peduase." And the designer said with the nodding of the head, 'Yes?' I asked again, "Where would I get the money and the plot for this?" The land where we were building was not big enough for the hotel and the only income I have is my little retirement and social security income. Then the designer said 'You will build a village'. "A village!" I screamed out aloud! 'Yes! You will also write a book.' "A book! How? Where and when?" I asked.

At this time the spirit took me to my hometown of Kwahu Aduamoah, Ghana, where myself and my two other siblings have purchased six plots of land about ten years earlier. These plots, the chief of the town, who is also a cousin, has been putting pressure on us to develop. The last I heard of the plots was a few years ago when it was brought to my attention that some people have started building on the property. Personally, I have given up on the plots. I know too that my other two siblings are not in any position physically or financially to build. I told the spirit, the designer, that I will talk to my cousin about getting the plots back. But the designer said 'No!' I said ok, I will talk to my older sister who is the reigning queen of the town. I know for sure she owns some lands, property of the clan or family. We, the family, have acres of land that we could use to build on. Again the designer said, 'No!' Then I was taken to the end of the town, where I stood on top of a cliff with the designer by my side. I was introduced to this vast evergreen land at the end of the town. The cliff marks the end of the township. One can see the continuation of the Afram Plains of Ghana. The Afram Plains surrounds or pass through the Kwahu area and that is what makes the whole place special and intriguing.

In fact legends have it that the Kwahus were in a fight with the Ashantis when the Kwahus ran up to that area and hid behind the gigantic plains and were able to defeat the Ashanti warriors whenever they attempted to climb to come and attack them. The plains pass through my hometown. It has this huge ragged tops, the greenery of which is so beautiful to look at and is a must see sight. My response to the designer was that I do not know if that property belongs to my hometown or to another township because the townships are so close to one another. The designer said, "Yes. You are going to build a village here!" I was still very surprised about the idea of a village. A village? Well, that vast land can surely build a village; maybe, even a whole township. So we stood on the hilltop and the drawings continued. The miracle of the whole idea is that I found out weeks later that that beautiful valley belongs to my family. I say that because the kings and queens of the town are from my family. My family stool is also the Kwahu traditional benkum stool. The custom is that the queen and the king are the ones to make decisions about land titles. This was true of all the towns in Ghana. In the past people used to say the town belongs to my family because of that and many other reasons.

My Hometown

My hometown, Kwahu Aduamoah, is nicknamed "Kwahu Bungalow" because it is a dead end town. One cannot pass through there by car to any of the surrounding towns, even though it is surrounded by other towns. There is only one entry by car and all cars that enter come out of the town the same route. Except for special occasions, the township is very quiet and the population is dwindling, another reason why it is still nicknamed a bungalow. To me, the town is slowly diminishing, no longer vibrant. People have moved away to the cities and big towns and only the elderly and their few grandchildren are left in town. The young ones come home on festive occasions only.

The town has a Catholic and Presbyterian elementary schools; an all girl's private high school which opened two years ago - the first and the only all girls secondary school in Kwahuland. I have been told not one single girl from the town attends the girls' school, even though the board of directors had promised full scholarship to in-town students. This is a town of less than two hundred population at any given ordinary day. The town has so many denominational churches. I heard there are eleven churches total; I always ask my family, whenever I visit, where the churches get their membership in order to survive.

The town has a market which opens once or twice a week, and a few small stores, including the one in my family home. Lately I see a couple of umbrella booths where one can buy telephone units or play the lotto. There is a town hall, and of course the palace needs repairs so badly. There is one river, Subri, which is the lifeline of the town - the only source of water supply for the town. The cliff where the Spirit took me marks the end of the town. From there one has to make a U-turn a few yards back. A left or right turn marks the junctions where one would be able to reach Abetifi or Obo walking. There had been politicians after politicians who have promised to construct a road joining the two sides of the T-junctions to the two neighboring towns, Abetifi on the right and Obo on the left, but those have   always been political talks. The moment the political party goes out of office the promise dissipates.

Kwahu Aduamoah is a small town well-known throughout Ghana for tiger nuts production. This small town has this special soil that produces the best tiger nuts to be found in Ghana. Throughout the ages, Aduamoah has been known for its farming and selling of tiger nuts. It is the major commercial crop. The youth, especially mature girls, secure farmlands and plant tiger nuts for commercial consumption. They take it to the big towns to sell after harvesting. Many I know got the capitals for their big businesses this way. All they required was to know or have an extended family member or a friend in a big city that can house them for few weeks while they go out daily to sell on the street, the African way. These are some of the ways they leave their towns and migrate to the cities, and they do not go back to live there except for occasional visits.

Conversations with the Designer (continued)

The designer said as a response to my question on where I would get the money to build the village, "You will write a book and you will use the money to build the village." Wow! Me, a writer? Well, to God be the glory! I said out aloud. Now! My immediate family has been urging me to write the story of my life, especially my love story since retirement and I have avoided it so far. So I thought of writing my story, my biography. But the designer said, "No, you will write the story of your illness. The story of your illness so people will know." I told myself that is a very grand commission but I am not a writer so how am I going to write a bestseller to make enough money to start building the village? This is when I remembered what my teacher at NYTS and my daughter Emi said in 2008. Ok! Again, the spirit told me I shall get help from people such as Oprah Winfrey, Maya Angelou, and Dr. Daniel Amen etc. Dr. Maya Angelou, I have known briefly and loved from afar since 1968 when I first came to America. She was one of the few dynamic black women who were Ghanaian-centric. She just loved Ghanaians. I only met her once that year. She was a dear friend of my brother-in-law, BB (Boateng Bediako). BB was the representative of the Ghana Black Star Shipping Lines in the USA. Their office headquarters was in Manhattan and BB lived at 706 Riverside Drive, Manhattan. Many parties were held there in the five-bedroom eighth floor apartment facing the Hudson River. I met Mama Maya Angelou that year on one of those parties at 706 Riverside Drive. BB left New York for Ghana in 1972, and passed away five years ago in Ghana. May he rest in peace and may his spirit continue to be a good angel watching over the family. I had planned to call on Dr. Maya Angelou, introduce myself and ask her for advice on this book when it is well on the way, therefore, her untimely demise in June 2014, the very week I returned from Ghana after a three-month stay, has been such a loss to me. Her death is an enormous loss to many and the whole world.

May she rest in peace!

I will take this opportunity to mention another Ghanaian-centric lady, Ruth Chiles, who at this time in the nineteen sixties lived and worked in Connecticut, New Haven. Ruth, who also passed away about eight years ago, singlehandedly was a mother to all the Ghanaian students at Yale. Ruth was a nurse and her house was an open door to all Ghanaians from the Yale campus. I met her through BB and she was a mother to me and my former husband. She was the godmother of our first born. I have lived in New York all my life, but Ruth was there at my wedding and all other important occasions. Ruth retired to Gainesville, Florida, where she spent the rest of her years with her family. May they all rest in peace and may they continue to be angels watching over us. Amen.

I did write to Oprah and tried her telephone contact, but a staff member told me my chance of getting to talk to her was one in a million. My last attempt was attending "The Life You Want" in September of 2013. From that time I decided to continue to write and see who God sends my way.

Chapter 15

The Designer at Work

The drawings by the spirit continued. This time the designer and I stood still on the cliff and the designer continued to operate to the left of where I was; and the drawings just kept on coming. We stood at the cliff for a while and before I knew it, the designer sketched out a city in a very large valley. A circular city the kind of which I have never seen. I asked the designer how one gets down to the valley and right away a tunnel and also a long set of stairs with side rails on either side was built on the left side of the tunnel. The designer started drawing with some strong, long, strokes on the walls down the valley. Again there was a large building with steps, windows and drapes visible inside the building. The drapes were so beautiful, very colorful and were being blown by strong winds. The long stairwells inside the building tell me this was a story building.

Then, scurry objects - which finally became furniture - started to appear on the ground floor. This was a story building because there were steps inside on the right side from the furnished room. I wondered if this was the beautiful tall building from the beginning which I first thought was a hotel when the visions started. This time the drawing was of the inside of the building. Again the miniature view of the city came to view. There were houses all around in the valley, small single homes with people busy going about their business.

Then we stepped back and there was a waterfall which kept on drying up underneath with large stepping stones. How can there be a waterfall with no spring to it? I said this to myself. I don't understand this. I had no idea if there is a spring or river in that valley up to date. The drawings for the waterfall went on for a while and it kept on drying up at the base and not becoming a stream. There was black and red soil on the ground between the stones or blocks. The vegetation was shrubby, wet and brownish on the ground. The scene showed only a stream that dries up at the end with a man-made passageway of large blocks of stones. Wow! Of course nothing made sense at this time. At this time it must have been about twelve midnight. The nurse came to my bedside and I complained to her that I have not fallen asleep since I was extubated post-op. I begged her if she could give me something to make me fall asleep. Her response was that she would check and get back to me. She came back shortly to let me know there was nothing for me to fall asleep. She added that there was a one-time order of Percocet for pain. I said I would take that because even though I did not have pain, I thought that might help put me to sleep. However, the painkiller did not make me fall asleep.

The designer continued with the drawings, with myself as an observer. A wooded field was shown down in the valley. The original trees were kept, some formed the fence or hedge to the field. There were so many trees forming a canopy, with the sun silhouetting through. The reflection of this was so beautiful I cannot describe it. There were benches under the trees, but I did not see any human beings on them at that time. This was a very large field. It had beautiful stone chairs, tables and benches. Then animals were drawn by the designer, one at a time. There were small animals like squirrels, rabbits, pigeons, mousses, rats and all kinds of small birds roaming and going in and out of bushes and the branches under those trees. I concluded that that was a park. But a very unusual park, a sit in park? A park with so many trees that gives shade and benches can only be a reading park, I concluded. There was only one clearing area and that was where the designer eventually sat.

We left that scene and went down to different parts of the valley. Then the drawings of big animals begun. There were big animals such as giraffes, tigers, horses, elephants, lions and all kinds of big animals. Some were in cages, which made me think of a zoo. Suddenly there were a whole township of animals; animal city? I don't know! The big ones were in cages and the small birds and squirrels just roamed about in and out of the trees playing. The interior of the circle of this village had several streets. Along the walls of this crest were small houses for human habitation. There were many small houses, all in the interior of the circle. More animals were drawn. Big animals in cages like in a zoo. Then the bigger houses were drawn with some scary figures which at this time were obvious to be animals or furniture.

A big house was drawn that looked like a theater. Then there were some animals with strings attached to them. I thought they were animals in a cage, but in the end a curtain was drawn and there were seats and pews in a large room. A theater was born and on the stage was something like a puppet show. Then there appeared another building with a screen on another site with an audience and dim lights. I assumed that was a movie theater. The most interesting part now began.

The drawings continued, this time about the people of this village or city. The drawings continued to be frightening at the beginning but eventually the end product was always exquisite. The end product was always something simple and familiar. The city was soon filled with people. Peasants selling produce in stalls, tourists buying and local people shopping. People walking with carts and bags, shopping. I say tourists because there were people dressed differently. Some wore different outfits or costumes representing different cultures. The scene was like a busy summer day in 125th Street in Harlem or 34th Street on Broadway in Manhattan where one meets people of all nations. Tourists or traders, they were all there.

Then the designer moved forward and this time he had on a beautiful long, multicolor gown with a hood and something like a kente shawl over the shoulders. I still could not see the designer's face, but the drawings continued. There were angels with wings and people dressed like angels with white outfits and no wings. There were people in the town's squire singing with small earthly angels and children and others listening and enjoying the music. The scene was very festive.

The expressions on their faces were heavenly. Pure joy and love. Their faces had such glow and their skins shone. This time the designer sat down on this gigantic or huge chair made of stone. Children that He drew sat in front and all around him.

I saw the designer's face this time. I have never seen any man that handsome, big and tall. He was a giant enigmatic figure of otherworldly origins. I mean a hunk of a man. His hair was curly, short and all white. There was something about him that makes you not to continue to look at him but just admire his work. So my eyes were fixed on what he was doing. Months later, as I write, I am still wondering what the city or village would be or what it will be called. To be continued.

Chapter 16

August 20th, 2013

On ABC morning news, I heard the bad news that the Vice President's son, Beau Biden, has suffered a stroke. The interesting question is why there has not been a great awareness about the genetic component of this terrible disease. The father, the vice president, has had a brain aneurysm with clipping at an early age according to the news. The news also says that the son, had earlier on, been suspected of having a stroke. My question is could this one have been prevented? What are we waiting for to start a massive campaign about the disease and making awareness and testing to prevent strokes? As a devastating family disease, stroke affects the whole family. Children, husband and wives, grandchildren and all loved ones are affected in a very bad way by this terrible illness. When are we going to tackle it heads on? I have already said a prayer and will continue to pray for his speedy recovery.

September 9th, 2013
The Designer Continues

It has been a long time since I sat down to write. The designer took me to the wall surrounding the community, the wall in the valley. Again the drawings began, but this time they were drawings of biblical figures. Few of them I knew, for example Abraham, Moses, Samson, David as a shepherd etc. These biblical drawings continued along the walls of the circle of the valley. There were important women from the bible such as the four Mary's in the New Testament: Mary, mother of Jesus; Mary Magdalene; Mary mother of James and Joseph and Mary wife of Clopas. Of course there was Martha and her sister Mary of Bethany. Then the drawings of all the Apostles started. At this point I told the designer that I will do an Internet search of the apostles, seers and the prophets and put them on the walls of the city. Again I told the designer I would take care of all the women and men by internet search.

Then the designer moved from the walls, moving slightly inside the center of the valley, leaving a space like a sidewalk and started putting up big poles, marble poles. On the big poles the designer started drawing again. I recognized Moses and Jesus. Then He began drawing a scary, fiery-eyed being. I became afraid and I said "Father, I am not worthy that thou should come to me, speak the word only and thy servant will hear." At this point I was thinking of God the Father, Son and the Holy Spirit. I was petrified. I was also thinking of the centurion in Matthew 8:8, who did not want Jesus to come to his house to heal his servant. He believed and had an unquestionable faith that all Jesus had to do was to speak the Word and so it was. I too had a strong belief that I would be able to find pictures of all the great people in the Bible on the Internet. I said once more, Lord, I shall check out the pictures on the Internet. The truth is that I was so afraid. How can a sinner like me look at God? I was unworthy. I just could not continue to look. I was consumed by fear, with just enough courage to say, "I shall do a homework with the Internet search?"

My nurse came to check on me because she said my blood pressure had begun to go up. As usual I complained of my not being able to sleep. She repositioned me in bed and encouraged me to sleep. I closed my eyes after she left and the drawings started again. This time there were people down in the valley, some walking, others sitting on benches. Some cars were passing. The cars were small bunnies, VW types.

This time the drawings were more complicated. The designer would start something like an object, like a flower, and the end product would be angels singing in the clouds or sitting at the feet of an apostle or some familiar great person in the Bible. I think this was so because I had asked the designer to stop drawing the apostles and other great people when I became afraid earlier.

Some angels were singing and others were playing harps, flutes and other musical instruments; further, some were singing with their hymnals, while others were dancing. They were beautiful and everyone looked very happy. I was happy too. I had no pain and every time I looked at the monitor by my bedside my vital signs were normal. I just wanted to sleep a little, but sleep was nowhere.

Post-procedure Follow-up
September 26, 2013 was when I was scheduled for post-aneurysm embolectomy angiogram. This was to be done on ambulatory basis. Preparation for this was simple. I needed blood work, which was completed and sent to my doctor at

August 20th, 2013

Weill Cornell Hospital a week earlier. The account on this procedure and the result will be discussed in later chapters.

Chapter 17

Back to the Visions
March 15-16, 2013

I continued to pray to fall asleep but sleep was nowhere. The drawings by the designer continued and I continued to be entertained into the early mornings, with no sleep. My normal routine of waking up at 4:30 a.m. told me it was time to tune in on the toll free conference line and join the praise team which would already be online and voila! I was the third person to call in that morning. In five minutes there were about ten of us online and I had a song that the team helped me to sing to praise God. The song was in Twi, my national dialect. It goes like this.

> *Medaa owu na, Yesu abeyang me (twice). I was in a deadly sleep. Jesus woke me up. (Repeat)*
> *Anigye a manya yi asee ne se,*
> *medaa owu na, Yesu abeyang me.*
> *Ayeresa a manya yi asee ne se*
> *me daa owu na Yesu abeyang me.*

The happiness that I feel, the healing I feel, the meaning is because I was in a deadly sleep and Jesus woke me up. By this time it was about 5 a.m. it was March 16, 2013 and there were about twenty people online. Majority did not know I was in a hospital, let alone that I had surgery. Every one of them thought I was in London taking care of my sick sister. I announced myself and I told them my trip was cancelled and that I was in a hospital. That I had surgery and I was ok but have not slept since 2 p.m. the previous day. That I was so happy and I wanted them to join me in giving thanks to God. They started praying out aloud individually as we do each morning during group prayers. I was using my cell phone. My nurse came to my bedside and said my blood pressure was up and that I needed to get off the phone.

Secondly, she told me I needed to be medicated instantly since my pressure has exceeded the required range. Of course I hanged up instantly. The nurse medicated me twice with IV. I was administered hydralazine IV to bring my pressure down. The designer continued with his work of drawings. I had the urge to call my brother's house in Washington to let him know my surgery was a success and that I am seeing things. I also wanted him to know that I had not slept since I woke up from general anesthesia the afternoon before. I actually wanted to talk to my niece 'Mama' whom I thought could help record what I was seeing. I could not remember Mama's major in college. I needed to be reminded of what she had majored in at college two years earlier. I needed to know if she was an IT major, in which case she could help me. And what do you know! Mama answered the phone at 5:30 a.m. in the morning. I should have known the designer was in control.

Furthermore, Mama told me her parents were asleep and so was everybody in the house. She asked me to hold while she gets a pen and paper to write. I told her I have not slept since I came out of surgery. That I have a spirit by my bedside telling me things I am going to do when I come out of the hospital. I asked her to start with the drawings as the designer was putting them out. To my surprise the designer started drawing pictures of my brother's household. My brother was the first who took a chair by my bedside, then his four daughters, including a diseased older daughter. His wife and all of their grandchildren were there. They were talking to me. My nieces were telling me to put them as some of the people in village. They said they wanted to be part of the village. In my room some were sitting and others were standing; the children were sitting on the sides and at the foot of my bed. There were only two chairs at my bedside.

Then the nurse came back with medication for high blood pressure because my pressure was high again. This time it was about 7:30 a.m. in the morning. The nurse tried everything to see if I could fall asleep. She gave me back massage and repositioned me side to side several times in bed but still no sleep. My brother and his family stayed at my bedside talking to me in the visions, telling me to listen to the nurse and stay away from the phone. His whole household and grandchildren were at my bedside. The faces were so clear, distinct and uniquely very pretty. I was just lying there calling each one by their names—even one daughter who had passed away nineteen years ago was there talking to me. Soon my other three sisters and a brother, their children and grandchildren were all at my bedside, singing and praising God for his protection. The whole African or Ghanaian extended family was at my bedside. I felt very happy. I was blessed and I knew I was highly favored by God. They made me realize how lucky I was, how blessed I was to have such a loving and caring extended family. All three of my Washington brother's living children wanted me to include them in the writing of the book and the building of the village. They were communicating with me in such a way that I understood all they were saying. The rest of the family members were just happy and were singing gospel songs, praising God. My brother was telling me to listen to the nurse and stay off the phone and stop talking. He sat in a chair at the right foot of my bed facing me.

There was a change of shift at 8 a.m. My nurse came to introduce the new nurse who will take over. I wanted to know what time breakfast would be and also added that I had not been able to fall asleep yet. My second nurse, who actually was my third nurse, was a male. As usual, I interviewed him in return and asked how long he had been in practice and whether or not he has cared for a patient who they claimed hallucinates as they claimed I was doing. He was sincere and answered no to my question. However, he promised me a different treatment. He told me my bed can be turned into a massage mode to massage my whole back by vibration from my shoulders to my feet. That was so wonderful. It felt so good, but still I did not fall asleep. Also, I was waiting on the breakfast which never came. The designer continued his work of drawing and talking to me and time passed away so quickly. When it was about 10 a.m. I decided to call home and find out when my daughter and husband would be coming to the hospital to visit. I asked my daughter to stop by the dollar shop on their way to the subway to buy drawing paper and be ready to do some drawings when she comes because I have not slept a wink since 2 p.m. the day before. I was afraid if I did not ask her to draw the visions I might forget everything. But fortunately they remained as vivid as they were the first day. She told me they went to my primary doctor's office when they left the hospital last night at 9 p.m. and did not go to sleep till after 2 a.m. She also added they will see me much later because they are busy cleaning and fixing the house for my post-op care. Of course she ordered me to try and go to sleep.

Soon after, my nurse came to my bedside and told me my daughter had called to ask him to tell me that I was not to use the cell phone because of the type of surgery I had. I called back between eleven and twelve noon to find out when they would be coming. This time she appeared upset because she said she told the nurse to give me a hospital phone instead of me using the cell phone. I called the nurse back and this time I asked for the bedside phone to be put on my bed, next to my call bell. Then I told him that I was told breakfast would be at eight and I did not have breakfast yet. I also enquired about when lunch would be. He answered, 12:30 p.m., apologized and added he would make sure I was served lunch.

The designer continued, but first my daughter called to make sure the hospital phone was accessible at my bedside and added that my doctor has discharged me to go home in the evening. He had told her I might be able to sleep better in my own bed. Therefore she added they will   see me in the evening. I was disappointed, I wanted her to come so she will draw my visions. I was afraid I might not remember everything. But I had no choice, so I closed my eyes and continued to talk to my maker.

During the morning several residents, both anesthesia and surgery, came to see me and there was not one of them that I did not tell I have not slept since I woke up from anesthesia the day before. Some of them said it has been documented on my chart that I have been hallucinating and others said it's my body's reaction to the anesthetic agent I received. I kept on hoping and waiting that my primary doctor will come so I could ask him. I needed to know why he did not prepare me preoperatively that I may go through something like that. However, he had told me the day before that he may not see me in the hospital before discharge if everything goes well. That he had left instruction for me to be discharged if all was well.

My nurse soon came and set me up for lunch. A regular diet. I ate everything on my plate. I had broiled fish, mashed potato and green peas. I also traded in my broth for another cup of jello. My throat was still very uncomfortable, but my appetite was enormous. I even sent my compliment to the chef as my tray was being taken away. I still had an indwelling Foley catheter and my nurse set me up comfortably after lunch to see if I will take a nap since I was still on bed rest with my intravenous fluid and all monitors in place. I have not had any pain since I had the procedure, just the lack of sleep. I was hoping that with my stomach full and comfortably set up I would soon fall asleep. I was not tired, and to my surprise, I could not wait to get to bed. I closed my eyes and started talking to the designer. During the day, from the time I talked to my daughter and husband, the visions were about my children, grandchildren and my husband's family at my bedside, singing and talking to me whenever I closed my eyes, while the designer continued to work, building the village. My family was very happy - my nuclear family knew about my surgery, but my extended family did not know anything was going on with me, especially those not in the USA. Thus, I was surprised to see the whole clan, especially those that I have not seen for years.

October, 5, 2013
Post-op Account (continued)

My daughter and husband did not get to the hospital till about 5:30 p.m. When they came, the nurse had sat me out of bed, dangled my feet and was about to ambulate me for the first time. Everything went well. I was sat up in bed, legs dangling and soon dinner came. I still had IV and Foley in place. My nurse said he would discontinue the Foley and get me up out of bed, and ready for my dinner. This was done with my daughter's assistance. Dinner was good. The visions continued with me sitting up. This time I could talk to my daughter and husband and tell them what was happening moment by moment. After dinner, I ambulated a couple of times in the area and was able to fulfill a post-procedure requirement of ambulating to the bathroom plus voiding. My IV was discontinued and all the ECG electrodes were removed from my body for me to get dressed with my daughter's assistance. The visions continued and I was able to talk to my daughter about what was happening every time

I closed my eyes.

The Journey Back Home from the Hospital

We left the hospital with me in a wheelchair at about 6:15 p m. The weather forecast on this day, March 16, 2013, was lousy. It snowed and rained all day and it was very windy. I had the back of the car to myself on our way home. I was supposed to keep my right leg straight. My daughter came with a pillow from home for me and I was in a lying position and very comfortable during the ride home. Of course the designer was at my side even at the lobby while I was waiting for my daughter to get the car. Weill Cornell had a fantastic valet parking system for family members who are taking family home after surgery. With my discharge papers, she came back to say it was zero charge for parking. I closed my eyes as usual and left my daughter in charge with her GPS.

The Drawings (continued)

This time it was mostly angels singing. The designer and I were no longer at the village. The angels soon changed to family members as soon as we left the hospital entrance and hit York Ave. From the hospital to the FDR is just a short distance and I started seeing strange things again. There was a car full of my family members ahead of us, behind us and on each side of the car we were in. The one ahead us was facing us and therefore driving backwards and there were cars behind it moving on. Family members in the cars were happy and singing. There was traffic congestion everywhere because of the weather. On both sides of our car, a great convoy of cars; there were cars coming towards us in front, besides and behind, but they were not hitting our car. I cannot understand how all five cars were moving abreast and there was smooth driving–one car did not collide with the other. All the people in the cars were singing and very happy. I knew everyone in these cars, my extended family with their children and grandchildren children. My immediate family was also all there. The cars on the sides were boom buggies.

The occupants in the cars changed the moment we crossed the Brooklyn Bridge. My family members disappeared in the cars and my church family took over. How that happened only God knows! Oh, what an awesome site! What welcome! They were all dressed in their beautiful cultural, national attires, the women with their big and beautiful hairdos. I don't think there was a face in that church that I did not see. Everyone was happy; singing and praising God. I kept on saying thank you Lord. I am so favored and blessed. They missed me and were so happy that I was ok, they acknowledged that. Both my family and the church family acknowledged and gave thanks to God. We were all singing praises to God. We met a little bit of traffic on Flatbush Avenue as a result of the rain. Fortunately the rain had stopped by the time we got to my neighborhood so I did not need help with an umbrella. My daughter assisted me inside the house, while my husband took out my belongings and went to park the car. The moment we got home I was assisted up the stairs into my bedroom and to my surprise, my daughter and husband had put a fall prevention precaution in place in my bedroom. The headboard to my bed had been draped with a comforter - a precaution to prevent me banging my head while trying to get in and out of bed. My room had been changed into an anti-fall precaution unit and set up for my comfort for the week. The discharge instructions said I should try not to bend the right leg as much as possible for the whole week.

I noticed my husband and daughter really worked hard overnight before they brought me home. The bedroom appeared clean with new beddings and drapery. I thanked God for their lives. They offered me something to eat and drink but I did not want anything. I was tucked into bed to sleep and my daughter went about her business to get herself ready for her one week business trip to Boston the next morning. She is quite a busy young lady isn't she, my daughter. I thank God every day for placing her in my life. She is such a great and huge gift that all my years of caring and nurturing cannot compensate. God bless her. This is God's grace. Amen!

Chapter 18

Visions (continued)

The Saturday night went the same as the night before with the visions. This time the designer drew someone whom I called God, under whose feet were angels singing. There were so many of them in such a beautiful, gorgeous oasis of a garden. A flower garden with every color, and flower represented. In this place, in this garden, were trees, flowers, staircases, a setting fit for weddings and happy occasions, and also beautiful and bright sunny blue skies. There were people with white robes, as well as angels. I asked myself, could this be heaven? Could this be the Garden of Eden or what? I don't have the words to describe the place. The designer was this handsome, giant, enigmatic man. All the men looked like him, but they were of normal size. Finally, I saw his face for the first time. There was this big man with a shining glow on his face. There was something godly and holy about Him, and I could see He had so much pleasure in doing what He was doing. There were women and men in all kinds of attire in that place. Each one of them was going about their business.

Occasionally I walked to the bathroom to urinate (pay water bill) like I do most nights in the past. Normally, I think my bladder is on a two hour maturation program. Few months earlier I went to see my doctor about that. I told him I have not been sleeping well because of my bathroom habits at night. My doctor prescribed a bladder medication called "Verised" which increased the hours from two to three, though eventually I stopped taking it. I went to the bathroom about six times that night. My husband, at least twice, asked me during the night if I have been able to sleep and if the visions have stopped. I looked at the time and noticed the time was eight o'clock and that I have dozed off for about one hour during the early morning hours. I told him I still have the visions. Anyway, I was able to sleep for an hour after spending more than forty hours being awake. On the third day the visions were not as intense as before, but they were still there. I was seeing more of my nuclear family and my church family who were mostly singing and dancing. I took naps in between the bathroom visits and eating. By evening on the third day, two church sisters who are nurses by profession visited and I told them about the visions I was having.

Sunday into Monday I had six hours of sleep with one visit to the bathroom. Eventually, the visions disappeared on Monday.

Two Weeks Follow Up Visit to the Doctor

The number one thing on my mind when I went to see my doctor for my two weeks post-op visit was to find out why I was not prepared preoperatively that I may be having these visions that they called hallucinations. I needed some sort of explanation. My doctor responded, "Ms Bediako, you are religious, right? You are spiritual and yours is my first case in my almost fifteen years of practice. They noted on your chart that you were hallucinating. I have been waiting for you to explain to me what all that was about."

Dumbfounded, I did not know what else to say. I wanted to know how many of his patients have shown such symptoms and judging from the above statement, the answer was "zero patients." He added that many years ago, about twenty years ago, most of the people that went in for this procedure with certain anesthetic modality woke up hallucinating. The anesthetic combination was changed and since then he had not heard of any further incidents. That explained why some residents at the hospital told me my visions were the result of my body's reaction to the anesthetic agent given. But I know better. I know what I saw, the village, everything. They were all created by the designer during those hours he was with me. I thank you Holy Spirit for Your vision. My visit was normal and I was given an appointment for three months' time.

My First Group Talk

During these three months, I had an eye checkup the third week post-op. The night of my visit I was awake in bed when I had a strong conscious feeling, like a voice talking to me; that today when I get to the eye doctor's office I should talk to the people waiting to see the doctor about brain aneurysm. I just responded "We shall see." I know that was one of the assignments the designer gave, but I did not know I had to start so early. My mission was clear: to preach the awareness of this devastating disease that continues to take our loved ones away. Surely when my husband and I got there at about 8 a.m. there were five people ahead of us and soon after the nurse came and opened the door there were sixteen people, with not enough chairs for them to sit. Dr. Agyemang was not in yet so I spoke to the nurse and asked permission to turn off the television for me to talk to the patients and their families who were waiting. Everyone was attentive, including the secretary. Soon Dr. Agyemang came and the talk continued. I was surprised how enthusiastic and attentive the audience were. They asked questions and others told of their experiences. Later when I went in to see Dr. Agyemang, he told me that he too has been listening and that what I was doing was a good thing. That was very encouraging. That gave me the confidence to give a talk wherever there is an audience and I get the spirit moving me to do so.

The next place I gave a talk was in my family doctor's office when I visited two week later and that too was a huge success. Dr. Wright liked it and encouraged me.

I made sure my neighbors opposite and on either side of my street knew about my illness. I talked about brain aneurysm and the damage it can cause if it ruptures. I talked to my friends at the park where we normally walk weekdays in the mornings between seven and eight in the morning. My audiences numbered between two to fifty people in the park. Everywhere that two or three are gathered and I got the urge to talk about my mission i.e. making people aware of the genetic aspect of stroke. Who in society gets the illness, the vast information available on the Internet plus how easily it is accessible was always the agenda, I never held back. I continued to give the talks wherever possible. Once at the Gethsemane Presbyterian Church at Park Slope, the reverend pastor, Pastor Diane Daisy, gave me a few minutes at the end of a Sunday service to say few words. At my home church I am occasionally given time to talk to the whole church or different groups. Meanwhile, I have been taking care of myself and I continue to enjoy life, thanking God every day. My family, church and friends showed so much support. I am so blessed that sometimes I can't contain myself with happiness. Meanwhile, I decided to stay in town till after my six-month medical checkup and possibly till my one year checkup before traveling internationally.

Chapter 19

A Setback
Small Bowel Obstruction

An unexpected complication or setback in my recovery occurred. Something terrible happened on May 13th, 2013. I ate something that soon after, I knew I should not have eaten. The baked plantain bread (ofam) was on my kitchen table for about three days in a foil. I should have refrigerated it. I woke up that morning and decided I wanted that for my breakfast at 8.30 a.m. So I warmed it in the toaster oven under bake. When I sat down to eat it with my first cup of tea, it tasted funny but I ate a small portion anyway. At about 10 a.m., I was hungry so I had this fresh beets, carrot and apple slush which had been in my refrigerator for three days. Of course my husband had been eating this slush for three days in a row. I love beets, but only when cooked or pickled. I decided to try the leftover beets combo slush. That was the first time I tasted that fresh vegetable combination, of course I have had borsch in my younger days. This slush was good so I enjoyed a full cup.

From that time, I was full yet at about 3 p.m. I ate a small boiled green banana and yellow squash/mackerel stew that I had planned to have for lunch. I ate half of the amount and at s6:30 p.m., my usual dinner time, I was not hungry but I warmed up the rest of the stew and had it with a baked small sweet potato, the size of a golf ball. All of the food eaten that day were leftovers. I needed to clean my refrigerator and what a nasty way to do it. My stomach became the garbage bin. Eating while one is not hungry is a sin and I should know better. My stomach started feeling queasy soon after that dinner. I went to the bathroom and got ready for bed after taking chewable papaya enzymes. The stomach pains started at about 8 p.m. and by 10 p.m. I had severe stomach pain with nausea. By 12 a.m. I had to induce vomiting by putting my toothbrush far down my throat. Then the vomiting started. I would vomit in the bathroom and by the time I try to get back in bed I had to go back. This went on until 4 a.m. By this time I became very weak and faint. I started moaning. My husband asked me if he should call an ambulance and I responded yes, but he had to wake my daughter up first since she was in the next room. When she saw me she asked to drive me to the NYM Hospital because an ambulance could take me to where my primary doctor may not be practicing. That was a very wise decision with God's intervention. NYM Hospital is where I used to work and we were there in twenty minutes. There was no other patient ahead of me at the emergency room. I was triaged and given an emergency room bed fifteen minutes after arrival.

The excruciating stomach pain and vomiting continued. A resident examined me and soon I was on my way to the x-ray department. The x-ray showed 'small bowel obstruction.' I knew I had vomited everything in my stomach during the night. I was still in so much pain to even comprehend what they were talking about. I just told my God that what they were saying was not true. I said to God, Lord, you just gave me an assignment, to build a village which I have not even started, how can I be diagnosed with such a hideous illness? No! This cannot be happening! It cannot be my portion! They tried to start an IV in both of my arms but it was unsuccessful. Two nurses and a resident tried but failed to insert one. A fourth person, a resident succeeded in a tiny vein at the back of my left thumb and then they gave me some antiemetic and morphine IV for the stomach pain.

Meanwhile, my daughter called my primary doctor as soon as I came back from the x-ray department to let him know I was at the hospital and have been diagnosed with small bowel obstruction. My doctor left word for a resident who normally follows his cases to see me at the ER and promised he would see me as soon as possible. His resident came to see me, and so did the whole team of doctors covering gastric patients in the ER. The surgeon on duty, not knowing I have a private doctor, came to introduce himself and told me I have a small bowel obstruction and that I might need surgery so he would be the one to 'cut me.' I thought that was crude and very unprofessional but I was in too much pain at that time to respond.

My family waited; they stayed at my bedside, refusing to go out even for branch. The nausea and vomiting soon stopped after I was medicated. I saw several of my former co-workers at the ER who spread the word that I was a patient and soon friends were visiting. I was assigned a unit bed right away and was soon transferred to a room. My family left in the evening after I was comfortably settled in my room. Dr. Wright, my primary doctor, came to see me in my room in his scrubs at about 8 p.m. He had just left the operation room and as late as it was, he said he had to see me first. He called my attention to the fact that his name was neither at the door nor at the head of my bed. Meanwhile he assigned a chief resident who had reported to him about my progress to see me. His resident also wrote my admitting orders. The doctor who came to introduce himself to me at the ER was listed as my primary doctor somehow.

Dr. Wright said that such incidents have been happening to some of his patients who present themselves at the ER lately. I told him his name was given to the receiving clerk at the ER at about 5 a.m., and also to the nurse at the triage area; therefore I don't know how such mistakes could be made. I told him that probably explains why the ER doctor came to make that weird introduction and proclamation. He smiled! He visited every evening and made sure the residents were taking good care of me and I never saw the ER doctor again once I was in the unit. My care at the hospital was good except for the initial confusion about who my primary doctor and surgeon were.

I was NPO (nothing by mouth) from the time I was wheeled into that emergency room that Monday until Friday night when Dr. Wright called me at about 8 p.m. from the office to see how I was doing. I told him I was a little depressed and he asked why. I replied that it was because the residents who came to see me this evening said that the repeated abdominal x-ray they took this morning still shows I have small bowel obstruction. Right away he said, "Agnes, let me call the x-ray department to forward the films to me and I shall call you back."

Dr. Wright called back in about one hour's time from the office. He said, 'I am going to disregard what the x-ray report says since you insist you had food poison; I want to try something different.' He told me he was going to call his resident to put me on a clear liquid diet in the morning and if well tolerated, he would ask him to advance it. He said he would not see me Saturday but would see me on Sunday. I took a deep breath and thanked God that at last someone has heard me. I told my nurse that my doctor said I could have a clear liquid diet in the morning and I had a good night sleep. There was no breakfast tray for me. My nurse had to get me tea and jello from the unit pantry. Lunch and dinner plus Saturday breakfast was clear liquid diet - broth, apple juice (which I hated) and sherbet. For lunch I asked for ginger ale instead of apple juice. You see I was very unhappy now because someone was tampering with my food! Don't forget the whole admission had been about food! Because I was a glutton for leftover food.

I was so happy when Dr. Wright walked into my room just when they served lunch on Saturday. He ordered me a full liquid diet for lunch, to be progressed to a soft diet for dinner. He also ordered for them to give me lactulose in the evening and at bedtime if I tolerate everything. He wrote an order to discontinue my Foley catheter and to discharge me home the next day, Sunday, if I have no further episode of stomach pain, nausea and vomiting. I could have danced with him if that was ethically possible. Everything went smoothly as ordered until the lactulose started purging me at about 9p.m. I continued in and out of the bathroom until I had no more to give. Between 4 and 5 a.m., I asked the nurse for a cup of plain hot tea with sugar and I was able to sleep a little after that. The good news was that I was discharged home in the morning with my pre- and post-admission sheet saying, "small bowel obstruction". I felt fine and walked home from the hospital to the car.

That was the miracle of the whole attack. I went to my doctor's office the following Wednesday and asked him how he normally treats food poison. In my case, he prescribed an antibiotic and also decided to put me back on Nexium for some time because at this time my whole abdomen was sore and very tender to touch. I was put on Nexium for about two months and I felt better. I continued to thank God for His protection and grace.

Through my writing this incident, I want my readers to learn this lesson that most of the time God gives us the wisdom to enable us to help the doctors He has put in our way to heal us. Again we should be careful of what we put into our bodies since there is consequence for every bad behavior of man.

Meanwhile I continued to give my talks on brain aneurysm and stroke wherever possible. August 11th was my big thanksgiving day at my church. I invited family and friends, in town and out of town, to come to church with me and on that day I gave my testimony to my church. A lot of my parishioners did not know I was sick. They thought I had travelled out of the country as usual. People were glad and thankful for the information. That gave me the incentive to go on.

On August 31st, my church choir, which I am a member, travelled to Toronto, Canada, for the choir's annual three-day conference. The choir consists of about ten or eleven churches in the US and one in Canada. The groups meet annually, with each church hosting once in rotation.

In Canada, I had an opportunity to talk to fellow choristers of about three hundred people, my biggest audience so far. I thanked God for that opportunity. I was not on the schedule, but the president of the group gave me a small window of about ten to fifteen minutes. It was such an honor and success that some members came to me later with questions.

Chapter 20:

Another Setback

September 26, 2013 was the day I was scheduled for my six months post-procedure aneurysm embolization follow up. This procedure would be an angiogram, which also required sedation. Two weeks before the day, my nurse practitioner had requested blood works, which I had completed and faxed to her at Weill Cornell. On that day, I was to check in as an ambulatory patient, after which they would do the procedure and send me home that very day.

But the devil was at work and strong. Both of my feet were hurting when I got home Sunday from church. I asked my son to massage both feet for me and went to sleep after that. Monday morning the left toe was swollen, throbbing and hurting. By Wednesday the toe was double the size. It was hot and pulsating. I could not walk on it. My nurse called to give me instructions as to where and when to report on Thursday morning. I told her about my dilemma, my swollen and painful toe. She wanted to know if I wanted to reschedule the procedure. I told her I don't know and that I would see my primary doctor that evening so I would get back to her. I went to Dr. Wright's office Wednesday September 25, 2013 with a cane and leaning on my husband. I was number four on the signed in sheet. By six thirty the office was packed. There were no seats for the patients and some were standing outside. Dr. Wright had not come to the office yet. Of course, despite my situation, swollen toe, pain and all, I seized the opportunity to give a talk on brain aneurysm/stroke. There were about sixteen patients waiting. It was one of the most interesting office talks ever.

There were two patients in the group who said they had suffered strokes and that they wish they had that opportunity I was giving others. One had a walker and the other one who appeared younger had her foldable cane in her tote bag which she took out for show. Each told their story and this younger woman said her stroke struck while she was on duty working in a hospital. She said she woke up after being comatose for days with complete left side paralysis. She had to learn to talk, eat, ambulate and do other activities of daily living. She said it had been five years since the incident and thanked God that she had almost completely recovered. She was lucky. Her attack happened in the hospital and she had immediate care. That is very important with this disease if one is to fully recover.

Others thanked me for sharing my experience with them. They said not everyone would do what I was doing in today's world. People are very private and they will not share their medical history with complete strangers. That was good to hear and it gave me encouragement and a reminder that what I am doing is one of the missions in my forty hours vision. It is not my doing but God's will, so we give him the glory; I am only a vessel to be used. We were so involved that the discussion continued after I had seen the doctor.

Dr. Wright was shocked to see my left toe. It was very

swollen, twice as big as the right. It was pale and hot. He told me upon examination that he recommends that I cancel the procedure at Weill Cornell. He could not find any previous blood work on the computer in which I had been tested for blood uric acid; just to rule out gout. The time was about 8:30 p.m. He said it was not possible for me to do blood work at NYM overnight and have the result ready for the procedure in the morning. I told him to give me the request form for the blood work and that I would take it to the hospital and ask them to do the blood work pre-op. He gave me a lab referral; and since we had planned to leave the house at five thirty in the morning to go to the hospital in Manhattan, I promised him I was going to ask my interventional doctor to do the blood test before I signed the consent for the procedure. This would mean that the report would be ready for me to get treatment right after surgery if needed. Dr. Wright agreed and gave me the referral.

The Six-month Checkup

Thursday, September, 26th, 2013 was a bright and beautiful autumn morning. We left the house at 4:45 a.m. This time my daughter drove. We had a smooth and safe journey. We arrived at the hospital early for my 7 a.m. appointment. I travelled with a cane because I could not put weight on my left foot. By 7 a.m. I was already on my pre-op/recovery room bed for my pre-op assessment. I told my primary nurse about my left toe dilemma and added I would only consent to the procedure if they would do my blood uric acid levels now. At first the nurse and the resident on duty tried to talk me out of my request, arguing that my procedure had nothing to do with the swelling of my toe. I told them my reason for the requests was so that I could call my primary doctor with the lab result post-op so he would call in a prescription to a pharmacy if needed. Luckily for me the test came back negative for gout. My uric acid was within normal limits. I praised God for that! Little did I know that after the procedure I would be instructed to have minimal weight bearing with my right leg! I was back in the recovery room and awake by 10:00 a.m. Post-operatively my right leg was immobilized for five hours in the recovery room. A complete bed rest, flat on my back for five hours, with right groin pain scale of 5-6 that I constantly refused to be medicated for. Wait! There was one thing very interesting this period. I had lunch. Lunch was served between twelve - twelve thirty. I was famished by the time the tray came and even though I was flat on my back with just a pillow support to the head, that lunch was the best meal I ever had. I had vegetable soup and for my hot plate was grilled tilapia fillet, spinach and mashed potato. I sent my complement to the chef! Then I was discharged home with instructions not to go up and down the stairs for a whole week again. Now I know I should have cancelled the procedure as my primary doctor ordered. How do I get home? How could the nurse and the resident tell me my left pulsating painful toe had nothing to do with my right leg? I was disappointed, but I was happy the procedure was over and that everything was ok. I was grateful and thankful to God and to the staff. I was thankful when my doctor came to tell me everything was perfect and that the clipping was effective; that I have had complete healing. God is good!

My daughter assisted me to get dress after discharge and I preferred to walk with my cane instead of wheelchair since I have been instructed not to bend my right leg. Besides I was happy to walk after lying down for all those hours. My left toe was still quite swollen, hot and painful. But the fact that the Uric acid test came back negative had a lot to do with my pain at that moment. I was also more concerned with the right groin, making sure there is no bleeding, swelling or pain at the sight. Soon we were home. My daughter drove us back home. I was assisted up the stairs at home and the routine was for me to be up there for the whole week. It was easier this time around. It was the same routine as before. Except this time I had left toe swelling with pain so the left leg was elevated all the time in bed while the right leg was to be kept straight on the bed. Unlike the first time, I had right femoral pain with constant pain scale of between five and six the whole recuperation period.

I thank God for my husband who waited on me, hand and foot for the whole week I was in bed while in this position. Thank you Kog! God bless you! This was the worst week of my life. Kog had to assist me out of bed whenever I had to use the bathroom or sit up to eat. I know it was not easy for him but God's love saw him through. By the third day we noticed a change in the swelling of the left toe, the swelling had gone down tremendously and the pain had subsided a bit. However, I noticed some weird rashes between the great toe and the second toe. They were painful rashes, hard looking and felt like shingles. But on the toes? I have never heard or seen shingles on the toes. I concluded I had an allergic reaction to some food, medication or bacterial infection. I went to see my doctor two weeks later when the rashes began to peel off and he tried to explain (something about a neural pathway that runs from the buttocks to the toes); believe me I cannot recall what he said but I was thankful my pain scale at that time was two.

During this time, Dr. Patsalides' nurse practitioner called to check on me and told me my next visit to the doctor would be in March, 2014. That was good news. Now I can start making airline reservations for all the trips I couldn't make earlier. Meanwhile I continued to talk to people about aneurysm/stroke awareness. Opportunities were everywhere, sometimes on the phone with friends that I have not spoken to since the procedure. People at the end of a conversation or talk would promise to get themselves or loved ones checked out. This has been my favorite pass time while waiting for my sixth month checkup and to make my first travel by air to Florida.

Chapter 21

Florida

The last time I travelled by air, I had such a severe earache on my to and fro Florida. That was during the Christmas holidays 2012 and January 2013. I did not have any ear plugs and the earphones given by the airlines could not help me. The pain was so bad I had to see an ear doctor on arrival. This time I had my earplugs ready the moment the plane was airborne and I felt no pain. I wonder if the aneurysm had anything to do with the ear ache. This is food for thought.

I was in Florida from November 2013 to January 2014 with my son, his wife and two granddaughters. Life in Florida with them was always fun. We went to Miami Beach, Kennedy Space Center, Busch Gardens and Disney. The children had Thanksgiving and Christmas holidays in between that time. I was there so we were always on the run. The weather was too cold for swimming but there were so much to do. I only did one to one talks about aneurysm/stroke awareness in Florida.

My Florida trip was to run from November 4th 2013 to January 4[th]2014. This was the time of the big snowstorms in New York. The week of my return flight to New York was a week that there were flight cancellations at Kennedy Airport. When I arrived at the Tampa Airport I was told the flight ahead of mine was cancelled because of bad weather in New York.

Our flight to New York was full to the wings as a flight attendant put it. We took off on time and arrived on time at JFK. On arrival, Kennedy Airport looked like a busy shopping center. There were people sitting or lying on the bare floors. People were running to their gates because their flights had been called the last minute. Twice I was almost knocked down by a couple and a lady running to a gate as I came out of mine. There were long lines for customs and immigration services. For baggage claim, we waited one hour thirty minutes before the luggage was put on the carousel. This had never happened to me. Thank God there were chairs to sit on while waiting. The airline kept on apologizing on the intercom. Eventually I was able to talk to about eight people about brain aneurysm/stroke at the luggage claim area. My trip to London was in three days' time, on January seventh. The airport was just as crowded because of the snow. I was in line with a boarding pass for luggage drop off, for one hour and thirty minutes, and the customs line was a forty five minutes wait.

London

Heathrow Airport was cool. All flights were on schedule. My pickup was outside with my name on a clipboard when I came outside after immigration and customs. Ben, the driver, was very friendly. He got the car and put in my luggage. It was a long ride from Heathrow Airport to my sister's flat at one Lesson Street in Brixton, London, so I had plenty of time to tell Ben about brain aneurysm, how it attacks more blacks than whites, more females than males and how the genetic component to the disease has been hidden. I also made him aware of the fact that if a mother or father have had stroke, chances are a sister or a brother will also suffer stroke, according to the American Heart Association. What had happened to me is frightening, but with adequate knowledge of my genetic history it probably could have been prevented.

I did a lot of individual talks during my trip to the UK. My sister was admitted to King's Hospital when I arrived in the UK. From the airport, the driver took me to my sister's ward for keys to her flat. In London, I talked to patients and their visiting friends and family. I talked to nurses, residents, doctors and other hospital staffs that came to the ward. This was because I spent at least four hours a day by my sister's bedside, seven days a week during her hospitalization. By the way, most of my sister's ailment had a lot to do with the fact that she had suffered several strokes since her fifties. Now she shakes so much that she needs help for activities of daily living. My sister, for years now, has to be assisted with feeding and bathing, and uses the walker at home for ambulation. For this admission she had gout and could not walk. My sister was also obese. This is my younger sister and she has been sick for so long and was on so many medications. The side effects of the medications combined had become yet another disease.

My sister had aged so much; strangers sometimes mistakenly think we are mother and daughter, while others say she is my aunt. That is the nature of brain disease. That is what brain illness can do to a person and to a family. I tell family and friends that the London trip was a working vacation. I put some work into putting things right in my sister's flat. There was so much junk to throw away and to put away. So much repairs and fixing had to be done by the Lambert housing unit. Hours were spent on the phone calling or waiting for repairmen to show up. In between, I spent time talking to strangers to look out for this killer disease. I was truly busy working. With all my talks in the US and subsequent ones in the UK, I realized people were dying for this information. I talked to people in taxis, as well as on buses and trains. I talked to cultural groups and anywhere one or two were gathered or when I had company. At times my traveling companions, namely my husband or son, get bored because it was the same talks over and over again. Sometimes I become embarrassed for them. However, I have a mission to fulfill so I keep going on. I say people are hungry for the information because after giving the talks, majority promise me that they were going to follow up and I believe them. This is my satisfaction and I am always at peace with my God, knowing I am doing what He had asked me to do.

I returned to New York at the end of January because I had dedicated the month of February for my medical checkups in preparation for my trip to Ghana, West Africa. First, I had lab works to complete and the doctor's appointments to fulfill. Every week was one or two appointments. First was the family doctor, then the Brain and Spine Center for my one year checkup since the brain aneurysm was clipped. For this appointment an MRI and MRA were done.

Chapter 22

The One Year Post-aneurysm Checkup
February 19, 2014

February nineteen, twenty fourteen, like the rest of winter days, was cold and snowy. My nurse practitioner at Cornell had arranged that I do the MRI, MRA plus see the doctor on the same day. At first I was given a 7 a.m. appointment for both at the imaging center, 416 East 55th St., then the center called me back after I had made transportation arrangement for drop off informing me that the technician and the doctor will only be in at nine. This, I told them, would affect my doctor's visit which had been scheduled at 9:30 a.m. fifteen blocks away. I told the technician to call the nurse back to explain and to reschedule the whole appointments plus call me back. This was done and my new times were 9 a.m. at the imaging center, and 10:30 a.m. at 305 York Avenue respectively.

My husband and I decided not to change the time for the drop off in Manhattan because of the weather so we left the house at 5:40 a.m. and arrived at the imaging center at six fifty. We thought it was wiser to be early than late due to the weather conditions. My tests were finished by nine thirty. We took a taxi to 305 York Avenue and we were on time for the appointment. Dr. Athos Patsalides had good news for me after reviewing my new brain Images. He told me everything was good. He said, "Now Aneurysm is no longer a factor for you. You have been cured. Your pictures show just a small dot like a blood clot". I said 'Hallelujah, it is God's doing. I give Him the praise, honor and the adorations'. Amen!

So I was given a clean bill of health except for the fact that my gait and clumsiness remained. Also my memory loss and forgetfulness remained. This, Dr. Athos Patsalides had warned me before the procedure that those symptoms may not go away. This is why it is imperative that we make awareness about the illness that people with family history of stroke will have checkups early. This way an aneurysm can be detected early and would not have caused too much harm by the time it is detected as mine was. We left the office about twelve noon for Brooklyn and I was in good spirit giving thanks and praise to God. This was my song in the car on the way back to Brooklyn.

> *Odo beng ni? (What is this love?)*
> *Awawa do beng ni? (What a mystic love?)*
> *Awawa do beng ni? (What a mystic love?)*
> *Odo beng Ni? d/c. (What is this love Dc)*
> *Me ne Jesu atena, (I have lived with Jesus)*
> *Mene no anantew. (I have walk with Him)*
> *Mafa Jesu se, (I have accepted Jesus)*
> *Madamfo pa. (My best friend)*
> *Awawa do beng ni? (What a mystic love)*
> *odo beng ni? (What is this love?)*

So, I sang this song all the way in the car and for the rest of the day. Actually I sang this song repetitively for several days. Don't ask me why, for I don't know why.

My next appointment would be an eye checkup which was scheduled for Saturday morning. Dr. Athos Patsalides has been concerned about my left eye since the procedure. He mentioned during my first post procedure office checkup that the aneurysm was too closed to the left eye (optic nerve) and recommend I see my eye doctor. I told him I visit one regularly and therefore I scheduled an appointment for each visit to his office. As usual my husband and I left the house early, at seven. Surprisingly enough, we got there at seven thirty and we were the first two patients that day. Dr. Agyemang was in at eight o'clock and we left the office before 9 a.m. My checkup was good. Dr. Agyemang told me that my eyes were ok. There has not been any change since my last checkup which was three months ago. I told him I have been feeling increasingly stickiness in the left eye. He explained to me that was the result of my eyes being dry. He asked if I have been using the ' dry eye' drops that he has been recommending. I confessed that I have not been using them. I promised I was going to start using now and regularly. Consequently I would say my checkup was good on that cold March day.

Chapter 23

Trip to Ghana

March 4, 2014 - June 16th 2014

My husband and I had our trip planned right after my annual checkup at Weill Cornell. I was given a clean bill of health. March in Ghana is very hot. I think it was hotter than usual this year. It was very dry also; the raining season was unusually late. New York had late winter and arriving in Ghana with khamsin (Harmattan) weather did not help me at all. Suddenly I felt sick. Both my legs were swollen. In fact I had first degree edema bilateral legs the first two months that I was in Ghana.

We stayed in my sister-in-law's house at Dansoman because our house that we were building at Peduase was not ready. Everything was good as always at Dansoman, and I was spoiled rotten by my in-laws. March is the month for pona (yams), so I gained about four pounds weight in about two weeks. I think this contributed to the edema of my feet. This was Easter time whereby I normally lose weight because of fasting or giving up favorite foods, but not this year. On March 17th my sister-in-law and I travelled to Akropong to visit the Presbyterian Prayer Center and also to see the evangelist in charge at the center. The honorable Rev. Dr. Abboah Offei was not available when we arrived at the hostel, but we were lucky for the presence of his assistant, Evangelist Dr. Asare who prayed for us and gave us an appointment to come back after the Easter holidays to stay for three days.

A Miracle in Ghana

As we were about to leave the retreat center, I asked Dr. Asare if a patch of greenery adjacent to the center was part of the hostel. His answer was "No, but Auntie Aggie you must see this." He suddenly started walking toward this place opposite the patch of land that I had asked him about. He invited my husband and me to follow. My husband was reluctant at first. He reminded me to be time conscious because we were supposed to pick up two grandchildren from school. There was this urgency about us seeing the place that we had no choice but to follow. Dr. Asare was walking so fast I had to instruct the driver to go get the car with my sister-in-law and to follow us with the car pointing to Mr. Asare, who was turning the corner by this time. Before my husband and I could breathe, we were standing at the Arboretum. It was a newly built prayer center and was not quite finished. He, Mr. Asare, continued to walk with us inward and it was there that I realized I was standing in a place similar to what I had described earlier as "Trom" during my vision. I realized I was standing on a Holy Ground. It was a miracle! I have never been to that place and yet there was this sense of "deja vu" about that place. There were some chairs circularly built in an area that had been cleared and new plants had been planted. In my vision the Designer was sitting in such a chair. How was that possible? I began to choke with excitement. I think tears started falling down my face. The place was cool so I would not say it was my perspiration that was on my face, despite the fact that I practically ran behind Evangelist Asare followed by my husband. This place was a ten acre prayer "arboretum" with a meditation chapel under construction. Wow! Behind the circular giant chairs were yams planted in small mounts all around. The place, which had acres and acres of land, had chairs and stone works for groups and individual meditation. I had so many questions for Evangelist Asare, but my husband was on my back about the 'time,' so I decided to save my questions till my next visit when I shall have the chance to talk to both evangelists.

The Grace Congregation, under the leadership of Evangelist Abboah Offei also dedicated a huge chapel and a manse on April 20th, 2014, an Easter Day function. I was there with some friends and family. After the Easter holidays I was able to visit the two evangelists in their office and get their full attention. I told them about my illness and about the forty hours that I could not sleep. I asked Evangelist Abboah Offei if he could help me build this village and he promised he would. In fact, he said my vision was an answer to his long time prayer. He had been praying that the Kwahu people get something like a prayer center, like the kind he had built. He was hoping to build a center up the mountains where people can go all year round to be with their God. The Kwahus spend one week annually to celebrate Easter. However, the way the Kwahus celebrate Easter these days has very little to do with the Biblical celebration. "Easter today as celebrated on Kwahuland does not reflect Christ's death and resurrection" the Evangelist said. Easter in Kwahuland is a one week affair. A time for family and friends to get together up the mountains. They now call it one week homecoming. Every Kwahu throughout the world tries to go up the mountains for Easter if they can. It is time for the rich and poor to visit the old folks they have left behind in their small towns. There are a lot of partying, drinking and frivolous lifestyle activities. There is robbery and people have recently lost their lives during Easter. We all agreed a retreat center for the village in my vision would be the most appropriate. For the first time the village in my vision started to make sense. Until that moment I just knew I was going to build a village. I had no idea what exactly the village would be used for until I saw the arboretum at Akropong. I know the village in my vision would have a chapel, a theater, a zoo, stores and vendor stands. The village would have a waterfall at some point, and a large hotel. A circular valley with small huts or shallots all around would also be there. The walls of the valley are to be painted with pictures of great men and women in the Bible. All of these and more were given to me in the visions by the Designer. But the park with all sorts of small animals roaming about, I had no clue that was to be part of a retreat center as I see now.

Meeting with the Extended Family

I started working on getting the land for the village by calling the elders in my family together two weeks later in Accra. I told them about my illness and the mission that I have been commissioned to fulfill. I made it clear to them that it was not my wish to build at this time in my life and that I am only a vessel to be used; and that I shall need their support. They were very supportive and they suggested we pay a visit to our cousin at Tema, who is the reigning chief, as soon as possible. We made an appointment right there and then to visit him four days after the meeting.

Nana Ohene Onini Afari the second embraced the idea with enthusiasm and promised to do all he can to help me acquire the land in question. He said the land in question belongs to me because it was the farmlands for my grandmother and her sisters. He even suggested there was some twenty acres of land which he had already demarcated for the Abetifi University Development but has not yet made it public. He suggested it would be mine if I want that area. Well, my answer was that the Designer picked the spot. So far, everything was smooth sailing and I knew God's hand was at play. I thanked the Lord for His favors, grace, mercy and all His blessings. The next phase was for me to visit my hometown, revisit the spot in the visions and to see the people who do the land surveys work in the town; who also can tell whether anyone farms in the area. This, by the way, was the hardest battle I had to face so far. The town committee is a group of people appointed by the chief, my cousin, to be responsible for all the lands in the area for purchase or for rental. Nana promised to speak to the local surveyor on my behalf before I talk to them. The committee met and found out that the area was an unmarked territory. However, the committee had to wait for the only surveyor in charge to come from his two weeks' vacation. He would work with them and his fees would be expensive I was told; estimated price for the mapping of the area was ten thousand dollars. I tried to lobby around with them by convincing them the whole project would be a humanitarian one that would bring jobs, good health and prosperity to the whole Kwahu area, especially our township. I called Nana back begging him to speak to the surveyor on my behalf. Meanwhile I continued to pray for a miracle and waited for the surveyor's return, while I celebrated the fact that the area the Designer gave me was an uncharted territory. Later my older sister, Queen Akumwah Sapongmah II, now the oldest reigning queen in Kwahu and probably the oldest in the whole of Ghana, confirmed the whole area belongs to our extended family. God is good!

I called a mentor and a friend whom I met at Akropong retreat center and asked my friend if he knew of any surveyor in Accra that he would recommend for a second opinion. To my amazement he did and I was able to meet the person he recommended the next day. This regional surveyor was more reasonable than the local surveyor that I have been waiting for to come back from vacation. The estimated cost for the job for the local surveyor was more than four times that of the regional surveyor. My immediate reaction was to let the regional surveyor do the job. After all I have not signed any contract with the local surveyor. However, my elders advised me to wait and talk to the local surveyor first, which I did. The local surveyor finally returned from his vacation. We met and I tried to let him know the project was a volunteer project, a humanitarian one; a nonprofit assignment and that I shall need help from everyone. He insisted he wanted the job, but for that higher fee. He convinced me that what he would do and what the Regional surveyor would do would not be the same. I wanted the local surveyor to do the job, but I did not have the amount he was requesting. Finally he agreed for me to pay in installment. I told him I shall be able to pay him the full balance in January, 2015. He agreed and promised to start the job right away. I did listen to everyone and though it was going to cost me four times as much, I thought it would be worth it in the end. I don't know if it was a bluff or not, but the word in town was that the town committee members can prevent any surveyor out of town from mapping the land. They would only allow the local surveyor to work with them. Here I was trying to secure a place for God's work, a land that I did not have to buy; but now confused because of the cost of the mapping. I prayed and gave it a great deal of thought then decided to let the local surveyor do the job for peace in the valley.

My Friend and Mentor: Another miracle

During the week that followed Easter, 2014 that I went to Akropong, I met a gentleman that I bonded with instantly. He was a young man in his forties. He gave me and my sister-in-law a ride from the Grace Chapel to the retreat center where we were all boarding. The encounter felt like we had known each other for a long time. I told him about my vision and I also told him my first born has the same first name as his. I asked him about his age and to my surprise, he and my son were born the same year. It was an instant love connection which I hope I shall have the privilege to talk about some day. After I returned to Accra from Kwahu I had an intuition to call my young friend above, which I did. I could not believe what he told me. He told me that he had investors from Finland who are ready to build a special surgery hospital on my plot as soon as it would be ready. That is a miracle, I could not believe my ears; I just had to say "Thank You Jesus. Already you are opening doors for me. First, a retreat center and now a specialty hospital, how lucky can I get?"

I know now that God's hand is truly at play. Thank you, thank you Lord Jesus for everything! We returned to New York in July for me to continue with my medical checkups and also to continue working on my book.

Back To New York

Today is Friday August 29th, 2014, I have made several phone calls to Ghana about the mapping of the land and so far the response has not been favorable. For this reason I am thinking of returning to Ghana soon. I left one fourth of the fees the surveyor requested with my sister, the queen mother, and she says the surveyor came for the total amount in June and had not paid the workers, therefore the workers are demanding for their pay before they continue the job. It appeared now that I made the wrong decision by letting the local surveyor do the job. I sent him a text message for the first time last Friday because he has not been answering my phone messages. He responded that he was going to resume work on the land this week. He also said he had asked my cousin, the chief, to talk to the workers. So, for now, all I can do is to pray and wait. He who started the project, I know, will bring it to a fruitful ending, that is my strong belief.

For now, I am concentrating on this book and also making preparation for shipment to Ghana after living in this house for over thirty years. Packing alone is a big job and I am not as strong as I used to be.

Lately I have been using brain busters such as ginseng, herbal supplements such as Brain Bio Boost Complex etc. My husband and I are both into special teas etc. So far, I have not come across that one special thing to give me the boosts of energy I need, but I am confident God will make the way. This is the final week of another Oprah/Deepak 21 day meditation, "Expanding Your Happiness" and as usual, it had been very helpful, very relaxing and refreshing. Thank you Oprah/Deepak. Today, Friday, August 29, 2014, I received a phone call from my brother's wife in Washington DC that my brother finally had an MRA of the head done and the doctor called back to schedule an office appointment next week because the report says my brother has suffered a stroke. This is the brother I commented on in an earlier chapter that I had been recommending for him and his wife to get tested. I asked my sister-in-law about herself and she answered me saying she did not get tested yet. I was very sad. I guess as the saying goes, a physician does not heal himself. I am not a doctor and I never claimed to be one, but I have this high intuition or feeling on certain things that one must carefully consider. It hurts to know however, that my family does not take me serious at times. I told them to get tested February 2013. I met them both in Ghana, March 2014, and seeing my brother and how much he had deteriorated confirmed my suspicions. I kept on calling them since we came back from Ghana until finally they told me they had scheduled an MRI of the head appointment. It took a year and six months to get them to go and see a physician. Who knows how much damage could have been prevented? I saw my brother March 2013 and again in March 2014 and he was not the same man.

I am so sorry that with all my talks of brain aneurysm awareness, someone close to my heart would allow such a thing to happen. But what can I do? We win some, we lose some. Such is life. We can only pray and ask The Lord to intervene. We are helpless without Him. I hope by the end of this week I would receive the full report and that it would be favorable.

First week of October 2014 was when my sister-in-law called to say that they have seen the doctor who said that the results were not favorable and that my brother recently suffered a mild stroke as I suspected. The doctor said my brother had the stroke as recent as three weeks before the MRI. This did not make any sense to me because I noticed a change in my brother way back in March this year. How could it be that the doctor says my brother recently suffered a stroke? My brother had been on warfarin since and the doctors have been trying to adjust the dosage.

Water Therapy

On October 2nd, 2014, I saw an orthopedic doctor for referral to physical therapy for bilateral knees pain. My arthritic knee pain has been getting worse and worse so I decided to do something about it. I started therapy October 16th. The following week, one of the Nigerian ladies who came to my house and prayed for me called. She told me how water therapy had been relieving her arthritis pain. Water therapy is simply doing aerobics or exercise in water. Through her, I found out that the New York Parks and recreations have recreational centers throughout the five boroughs at very reasonable rates, especially for senior citizens. These centers are equipped with pools, basketball and tennis ball courts and above all, the largest equipped exercise room with thread mills that I have ever seen. The place had large conference halls and other activity halls available for members only. They have educational programs such as free computer training, swimming, aerobics, aikido, GED etc. Naturally my husband and I joined the next week and though I continued with the therapy for four more weeks, I quit as soon as my six weeks were up. I have been going to the center since mainly for water therapy.

"The Life You Want Experience"

Meanwhile I continued to talk about brain aneurysm to groups and individuals. In September, I had the pleasure of attending Oprah's "The Life You Want" in Jersey City, Newark. That weekend was a thrill for me. I got to talk to several of Oprah's team members at the "O Town". I also got the thrill of giving individual talks to other attendees, whether over lunch, breakfast at the hotel or in the stadium. I noticed this weekend that it would be very difficult to contact Oprah so I decided to continue on my own and see what God will do.

Almost all the time, I talk to cab drivers taking me to and from about brain aneurysm, strokes and the hereditary component of the illness. I get great satisfaction when I am at the end of my destination and they are still asking questions and are very grateful. I tell them the thanks belong to God. Each year in November, the week before thanksgiving, the North American group of my church meets for a retreat with team members from Grace Prayer Center, Akropong, Ghana. They always come with their leader and his assistant, Prophet

Dr. Abboa Offei and Evangelist Asare. These two men of God are my mentors. Every year church members from USA and Canada spend a week in retreat with them at Stony Point or Keswick retreat center for prayer, worship, deliverance, giving thanks and dedication services. I was not able to join them this year but my church was lucky to have them administer to us for four days before they left to go back to Ghana. I had the privilege of being on one to one basis to talk to them both about the Aduamoah project, knowing for sure that they are both behind me one hundred percent with their prayers and support.

During this same time I had confirmation that the mapping of the land for the village was completed and any project on the land could be started. I wanted to make sure of a proper start, so I started increasing my effort to go back to Ghana to make sure that the land is registered both centrally and regionally. I have quickened my effort to pack and ship my belongings to Ghana and I hope I will be able to do so by January. Right after my birthday, in December, I came to Florida to spend the Christmas and the New Year with my son and his family. This was a big vacation for me from working so hard packing in New York. It is my wish that God will grant me the energy when I go back to have everything ready for shipment in two weeks. My house goes on sale after shipment because I plan to spend most of my time working on my vision, which is my mission until my Savior calls me

CHAPTER 24

A Donation for Ghana

Letter to Doris Sintim-misa in the Name of Sankofa

I returned to New York, freezing, snowy weather, just so I can continue to complete the packing for shipment. The next day my daughter Doris visited and saw me struggling to pack. I told her I needed more empty boxes and she told me she could bring me some. I also learnt from her at the same time that her hospital has some expired disposable syringes for donation. Right away the volunteering spirit in me awakened and I asked if my nephew and I could write a letter so as to receive the items, add them to my shipment and donate them to some Government hospitals which I know are struggling at the Kwahu and Accra regions. A letter was set in motion and Atibie and Tete Quashie hospitals will receive a large portion of hospital supplies when the shipment arrives in Ghana. These supplies were in their original cases and in very good condition. In America they are disposable, but in Ghana most of them are reusable. The packages delivered were in small boxes and I had to put them into big boxes. There were syringes, needles of all gauges, ambu bags, thermometers, dressing pads, suture removal kits and all sorts of disposable equipment that these hospitals in Ghana need so desperately.

Monday, January 12th, 2015, I had lab works at New York Methodist. The weather was predicted to have rain, be windy and cold, with snow coming later. The lab was not busy so my husband and I had quick service. The rest of the morning was supposed to be spent receiving donation supplies for the hospitals to be added to the shipment, though the event was cancelled because of the weather. I thank God for that because I was very tired that day.

Today is Friday January 16, 2015. I have been up early packing. I was expecting a repairman and delivery from the hospital. My doorbell rang at 12.30 noon and there was Doris with her car full of syringes for the hospitals in Ghana. Soon my living room was packed full with boxes. There was no place to sit. I had not finished packing my personal belongings in order to accelerate the shipment. In fact this would be the second time that this small organization, Sankofa, has extended its wings to the motherland Ghana through me. The first was in the form of a check for $3,000.00 (three thousand dollars) to Korle Bu in 2003 to help HIV victims. So this time we are going to the mountains. Praise God, hallelujah!

Mr. Alfredo, my repairman, came soon after Doris left for work to fix my storm door to the main entrance. I had to explain to him why my living room was full of packages and right away I started with my advocacy talk about brain aneurysm awareness since this was the first time we met. I talked to him the whole time that he worked about stroke and its devastating effect on the family once a member suffers it. We talked about whom, and at what age one may be a candidate for brain aneurysm; we also talked about the effect of bad habits and poor diets as some of the causes. The hereditary component was emphasized of course. The job took longer than expected. Before I knew, two hours had passed and I too had been on my feet packing and talking to Mr. Alfredo. At the end of this time Mr. Alfredo was treated to lunch. A Ghanaian cuisine of plantain fritters, some brown rice and good old beans stew. I can tell I made his day, and in the end he expressed his enlightenment about brain aneurysm and stroke. The job was not cheap, and my husband expressed that that was the most expensive talk I have given yet on brain aneurysm and stroke.

Chapter 25

April 1, 2015

Today is when I went for my two year post-brain aneurysm embolization checkup. I had it done at Weill Cornell Radiology department and I saw Dr. Patsalides right after the test. He told me part of the report was in and so far everything looked good. He said the rest of the report should be in the next day and that they will call to give me the full report. He added that he was pretty sure all will be well. He wished me 'Bon voyage" in advance on my trip to Ghana. I did not hear from them the next day till about four thirty p.m. when the nurse practitioner called to tell me the findings were not clear and that Dr. Patsalides would like to schedule me for an angiogram just to make sure that what the MRA shows was not a refill of the stent. This was a big blow to me, a big setback because this was the very week I purchased my ticket for Ghana and all has been set for my trip to Ghana. With that phone call, I wanted to know if a re-clipping or re-embolization could be done at the same time as the angiogram if needed and the nurse could not assure me of that. She said the doctor was on two weeks' vacation and would like to do the procedure angiogram as soon as he returns. I had told them I was going away for a long time so she said the sooner the better. So we scheduled me for the 14th of April, 2015. Meanwhile, I told my daughter who, of course, wanted me to get a second opinion before any further procedures. Search for another interventional radiologist was not easy. My doctor was away on two weeks' vacation and the one I found at Columbia Presbyterian was also not available for the next three week; he would see me on the 22nd of April.

Dr. Athos Patsalides had his nurse schedule me for the 14th of April, the very day he returns from vacation. Again I went to see Dr. Albert Wright and he told me not to worry and that he will call and speak to the nurse practitioner and if there was any way he, Dr. Wright, could text my doctor to find out what was going on, he would. At the same time Dr. Wright requested for the report of the MRA from the nurse. Meanwhile I went to the radiology place in Manhattan, Cornell, to pick up a CD report of all the radiology works that I have done there. This, Dr. Wright said he would show and discuss with some neurologist he knows and see what their recommendations would be. Again the second consult required that my primary doctor faxed all my medical history and any previous report relevant to the aneurysm, as well as bringing the report and the CD.

This is "Deja vu", I cancelled a London trip the first time I had the embolization in 2013 and I only purchased this ticket for Ghana two weeks ago after months of procrastination. I know this requires God's intervention, so I kept on praying and meditating, of course with Oprah/Deepak. This was the middle of another 21-day meditation titled, "True Success". I also continued to talk to my God, telling Him He is in control. Of course this was the Resurrection week, the week of Easter, the first week of April, 2015 and I sang and prayed for the resurrection power of the Lord to heal me as I waited. Dr. Patsalides returned from vacation and I had called the nurse to tell her I was not going to have the procedure until I speak to him. I did not hear from him until Monday, April 20, 2015. He called to explain to me the need for the angiogram. I told him since angiogram is an invasive procedure, I would like to be prepared for the re-canalization just in case. I asked about blood thinners and he ordered Plavix po and changed the time for the procedure to Friday April 24th. Of course that gave me ample time for my second opinion. Meanwhile, my medical clearance, blood work, chest x-ray and EKG report had all been faxed to their office for a Friday procedure just in case.

The consult with Dr. Sean Levine at the Columbia Presbyterian Neuro Center went well. My husband and I were late as a result of transportation delay and heavy traffic from Brooklyn to Manhattan, but Dr. Levine waited for us. The secretary took the CD of my radiology record from Cornell to him the moment we got out of the elevator. Dr. Wright, my primary doctor, had also faxed the forty paged file of my aneurysm history to the office the week before. Soon we were called in and Dr. Levine made us feel at home. They even had me down as a faculty member. The secretary told me I was in their system as such since I used to work there and that she was only going to update my chart for the consultation. I worked at Columbia Presbyterian Hospital full-time status, Med–Surg., 1983-1984. I have not gone back there since that year. This is grace as the Lord gives, and I am thankful to the Lord.

Our visit with Dr. Levine made me feel better. He asked me if I knew whether my doctor at Cornell used one or two pipelines for my stent, I told him I did not have that information. Then he looked in my chart and read the doctor's notes and confirmed that only one stent was used in my case. Dr. Levine said Columbia uses two tubes these days because two is better to prevent early bleeding. He said he has had patients with post-procedure bleeding like me whom he observed for a couple of months and then repeated the MRA and sometimes he did not have to go in for further re-canalization. My husband and I asked questions and I must say I felt confident that I could go to Ghana and come back safely before any further intervention. From Columbia Hospital, we took the Limited bus to our favorite restaurant downtown Manhattan for lunch and took the train few stops to Dr. Wright's office. It was 4:10p.m and there was no place to sit in the office. He was already serving #7 and I signed in as #24. The evening went fast. We were called in by 6:00 p.m. We told Dr. Wright about my consult and he was pleased about Dr. Levine's diagnosis. He promised to call Dr. Patsalides in the morning to discuss with him the possibilities of me going to Ghana for a couple of months and coming back for a repeat MRA or angiogram. That relieved some of my stress. Thursday morning came and went with no phone calls, then the nurse practitioner called me at about 1:30p.m. to give me pre-op instructions and where to report to Friday morning. I told her that I would like to speak to Dr. Patsalides first and that I have almost decided to go away and do the procedure on my return, but first I would like to know what my doctor thinks about the decision. She told me the doctor would be tied up in there all day and may not get to me till about 9:00 p.m. So she gave me the instructions and said she would be in until 5:00 p.m.

Dr. Patsalides called me about 2:30 p.m. He said he could not call Dr. Wright because he was in between cases in the OR. I told him how I was feeling and asked if it was ok for me to go to Ghana for a month or two before consenting to the angiogram. He said it was not ok with him and therefore I would be travelling without his consent. I told him I know for sure that I will be ok and that I shall call him as soon as I come back for further consultation. One of my nephews called me to find out the events of the day. He was happy when I told him I did not consent to surgery and that I will take my trip as planned. He told me his best friend who suffered stroke in April 2013 is in the hospital with another stroke. He said it was bad again. In 2013 the friend was given a 20% chance of survival and through love, prayers, patience, dedication and perseverance, he had recovered to 90%. Every one of us was happy for him and his family and now this? I said a short prayer and I said "Father, I do not understand". A song "Kyere me Ase Me Wura" (Father explain this) came to mind as I fell asleep.

My nephew was going to visit on the morrow, Saturday. I asked him to pick me up so I can visit with him. We left my house 9:00 a.m. with his thirteen-year-old daughter in the back to go to New Jersey to pick up his twelve-year-old son and then we would drive back upstate New York to attend a first communion of the friend's nephew to be followed by a party for the kids. There was so much traffic on the way that we did not get to the son's place in Orange County, New Jersey till 12:14 p.m. so we missed the church service. We made it to the reception upstate at 2:30 p.m. The plan was to take the sick friend's two sons to visit their father in the hospital, but the children decided they would rather stay for the day. So the hospital visit did not happen. Maybe it was for the best. I got home very tired but in one piece about 8:00 p.m. and went straight to bed. It is 11:00 p.m. and I am already awake and writing. I cannot sleep any more. I have too much on my mind. It is scary to know that the aneurysm can return as early as two years; especially with my nephew's friend back in the hospital. So I sang a verse from one of my Anglican hymnals that I still remember from the 1950s:

> *What shall I render to my God?*
> *For all His mercies given,*
> *I'll take the gifts,*
> *He has bestowed,*
> *And humbly ask for more. Amen!*
> *Eye Adom Nkutoo! Thank you, Father, Jesus.*

Chapter 26

Conclusion

I woke up Monday morning, April 27, 2015, for my morning devotion online. The scripture lesson today was Genesis 47. My pastor, Rev Dr. Moses Biney was leading the 30 minutes Bible study. A brief review of last week's sturdy took us back five chapters on the life of Joseph, how God predicted or revealed to him in a dream as a child that he will be great among his generation. How the brothers hated him for their father's love and his big dreams and how our Lord came true with His promise. Now Joseph told his brothers that he had forgiven them for their evil acts and that God intended for him to be where he was at that time, in Egypt as Pharaohs number one man, for their sake. That was an Aha! moment for me! The act of forgiveness and love. The act of humility and kindness, caring for the other person instead of oneself and the act of compassion all manifested itself in Joseph's kindness and love towards his brothers.

The song that came through was "Onyame Anuoyam Beda Adi" (God's grace would shine or manifest itself):

Onyame Anuoyam Beda adi o
Ama Amang, Amang nyinaa ahuse
Eye ono Agya Nyame na Waka se
Obeshyira yeng ama yaye Nhyira!

The above Ghanaian Gospel song is literally saying that God's glory will manifest itself, no matter what. Whatever the Lord has destined or ordained on our behalf would definitely come to pass. We are vessels to be used by Him to bless others while we are on earth. The big question is, are we a blessing to others? Are we living up to our great potentials? How is your human experience so far, my good sister and brother? Are we good shepherds like our Lord and Master? The creator God, who created us in His image?

This book is about the human brain and my experience as I battled with the illness of brain aneurysm and mini strokes. Nothing is impossible by God. God might take a long time and we as humans must learn to trust and obey plus believe in Him with humility. I just know because of the scripture reading that came through today, April 27, 2015, that God wants to use you, my reader, and myself to be a blessing to others. I know this as my mission for sure. My next book, which will include part of my life story, will talk in detail about my childhood, some of the benevolent associations that I have been privileged to be involved with, both here and in Ghana, and how God had used me to be a blessing to others. The proceeds from these books would be used to build an international village with a big meditation center, a hospital, farmlands, and a board walk at the Graceland at Kwahu Aduamoah. I hope you will join me in making this vision a reality.

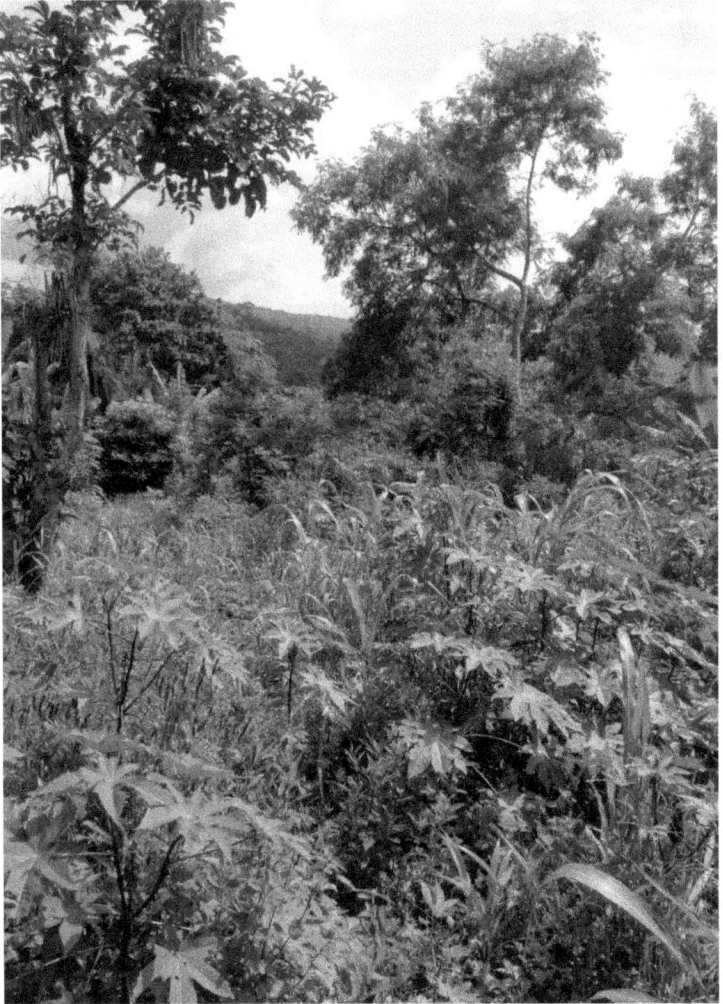

I thank God that He deemed me worthy of a call. I see the call "to build a village" as bigger than life. Our God is good, awesome and great. Amen.

Conclusion

Thank you for your support of purchasing this book, God bless you.

BIBLIOGRAPHY

Amen D.G., M.D. *Change your Brain, Change your Life. ISBN 0-8129-2998-5*

The Brain Aneurysm Foundation

www.bafound.org/unruptured-brain-aneurysm

"www.webmd/brain aneurysm topic overview. Jan 2011".

WebMD Medical Reference from Healthwise, January 03, 2013.

Brain Aneurysm: causes, Symptoms, Diagnosis, and Treatment - www.webmd.com/brain/tc/brain -aneurysm-topic-overview? page=3 rdsk=active.

Johns Hopkins Aneurysm Center: Unruptured Brain Aneurysm

thenationonlineng.net
www.derby.anglican.org/attachments;